CANINE *Massage*

A Complete Reference Manual

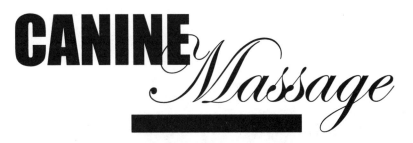

2nd EDITION

Jean-Pierre Hourdebaigt, L.M.T.

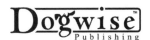

Dogwise Publishing
Wenatchee, Washington U.S.A.
www.dogwisepublishing.com

Canine Massage — A Complete Reference Manual, 2nd Edition

Jean-Pierre Hourdebaigt, L.M.T.

Dogwise Publishing
A Division of Direct Book Service, Inc.
PO Box 2778
701B Poplar
Wenatchee, WA. 98807
509-663-9115/800-776-2665
Website: www.dogwisepublishing.com
Email: info@dogwisepublishing.com
Graphic Design: Anderson O'Bryan, Wenatchee, WA

Limits of Liability and Disclaimer of Warranty:
The author and publisher shall not be liable in the event of incidental or consequential damages in connection with, or arising out of , the furnishing, performance, or use of the instructions and suggestions contained in this book.

Library of Congress
Cataloging in Publication Division
101 Independence Ave., S.E.
Washington, D.C. 20540-4320

Library of Congress Cataloging-in-Publication Data

Hourdebaigt, Jean-Pierre.
Canine massage : a complete reference manual / Jean-Pierre Hourdebaigt.– 2nd ed.
  p. cm.
Includes bibliographical references (p.).
  ISBN 1-929242-08-5 (pbk. : alk. paper)
1. Dogs–Diseases–Alternative treatment. 2. Massage for animals. I. Title.
  SF991.H596 2004
  636.7'0895822–dc21   2003010793

Printed in U.S.A.

TABLE OF CONTENTS

PREFACE

Life is a constant process of learning that brings deeper understanding and appreciation of one's skill. The inspiration for this book originated with my first experience with canine massage more than 20 years ago. Since then, I have had the privilege to share valuable information with many other canine professionals as well as with the students who attended my hands-on practical sessions.

It thus seems appropriate that I should bring you this revised edition with new and valuable information to better assist the on-going development of your educational process. My goal is to help you improve your skills and provide you with a deeper understanding of this beautiful and amazing trade. The study of this new material will aid you in recognizing the various musculoskeletal problems your dog might have, and the application of what is learned will produce rewarding results for you, the conscientious dog owner, and your dog.

Today the overall benefits of regular massage are better understood and appreciated and consequently the application of canine massage is becoming more widespread and accepted. Increasingly massage professionals, as well as dog owners, are getting involved in helping their canine companions through the application of gentle massage sessions. Regular massage not only provides many benefits to your canine friend, but it gives you precious indications on his overall fitness. This valuable tool will enable you to better monitor the growing dog, the dog in training, the dog in competition. and even the elderly dog.

This book is not intended to be used as a substitute for medical advice of a licensed veterinarian. Rather it is designed to give practical assistance to the dog owner or any professional to better cope with the everyday situations in the life of our canine friends.

Regular massage applications create a great bonding experience between you and your dog. One of the most valuable and pleasurable experiences in my life has been to see this book bring great satisfaction to both dogs and owners. I hope you too will benefit from it.

Jean-Pierre Hourdebaigt, L.M.T.

DEDICATION

To my wife Brigitte whose support,
patience and love made it all possible.

ACKNOWLEDGEMENTS

To all dogs, thank you for making me smile, for sharing your stories, needs and secrets, and for inspiring me to write this book.

To the dog lovers and dog owners—my gratitude for your years of participation in my seminars, for sharing your knowledge, for giving me your feedback, support and encouragements. Like your dogs, you have been a source of inspiration.

For making this publication possible, I thank: **Brigitte Hawkins**—for her knowledge and talent, her desktop publishing and photography skills; **Janet B. Van Dyke**, DVM and **Jim Berry**, DVM—for contributing to and verifying the medical content of this text; **Shari Seymour**—for her talent in preparing the illustrations used in this book; **Cleo and Casper**—for their modeling talents, patience and their enduring sense of humor.

The Dog and Massage Therapy - An Overview

In preparation for massaging your dog, it is important to first put yourself in the right frame of mind. Besides your knowledge of the dog's anatomy, physiology, and all the massage techniques, to get the best results from your work you need to give your full attention to your dog. By being fully attentive you will be better able to feel the structures of the dog's body and assess his needs at the time of the massage. Put aside your personal concerns or worries so you can completely involve yourself in the work. Do not start when you are stressed, anxious, tired or fearful. Your feelings will be passed on to the animal through your touch, so be relaxed and have a positive attitude. In other words, the way you are is the way the dog will be. If your mind is not on your work, it will reduce the quality and effectiveness of the massage and your dog will be the first one to notice.

Consider the "ambiance" of the room where you will be giving your dog his massage. Perhaps dim the lights, play soft music. This preparation will help you make the transition and prepare you for the massage. Indeed when you first begin you may feel a little hesitant about giving a massage, but with practice you will quickly overcome this feeling. As long as you truly connect with your pet during the massage, he will feel cared for and that is most important. Another consideration is that if you want to know how it feels to be massaged, contact a licensed therapist in your area and treat yourself to a full body massage, preferably a Swedish massage. You will be able to experience what I term "feel-see" first-hand the various massage strokes that are taught in this book as well as the routines and techniques, the relaxation, the caring feeling, and the depth of work that massage can provide. Then you will better understand the effect you produce on your pet when you deliver a massage.

Approaching the Dog and Initial Contact

Your first contact, the actual first few minutes with the dog, is crucial for the positive development of the massage. Dogs, like humans, will sud-

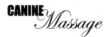

denly tense up if they feel their bodies are being invaded. It is crucial you develop some trust between you and the dog you massage. I recommend that you observe the animal carefully before starting. If you approach the dog with an understanding of its realm and immediately make it feel secure, your dog will develop trust in you very quickly. Remember your dog needs to be "massage trained". Use positive reinforcement by praising and rewarding your dog when he acts appropriately. The situation requires awareness, some common sense, and a lot of dog sense.

Speak softly and kindly to the dog as you approach him. Present your hands fully opened. Do not move your hands too fast. Give your dog time to acknowledge you before you start. The dog's response will be to bring his head towards you and nuzzle you—this is how a dog shakes your hand. Meanwhile, evaluate the breathing rhythm and adapt your breathing to the dog's. This action will allow you to observe the inner state, whether calm or restless.

Once the dog has acknowledged you, quietly bring your right hand—your natural giving hand—to the nose and lightly massage the face (muzzle, ears, back of the head). Keep talking and praising your dog, furthering your bonding with the softness of your voice. Gently bring your left hand to the dog's attention, then start touching the neck lightly, at the back of the head. If the animal does not like this, bring your hand down to the withers.

The first hand contact needs to be very warm, thoughtful and rich in feeling and vibration, so this contact will have a strong, positive impact on the dog. Be smooth. There is no need to rush. A few minutes is all it will takes to establish this crucial first impression. Keep your voice gentle and praising as your dog accepts this first massage contact. The relaxation routine discussed in Chapter 7 is the best way to start any massage session, especially if you are breaking the ice for the first time.

Maintain verbal contact with your pet—praising or commending as needed—as you progress in the session and look for feedback signs from your dog. Memorize the four "Ts": Temperature, Texture, Tension and Tenderness (see Chapter 4). Your fingertip perceptions are very important; ensure that you are mentally connected with them at all times. Take notes of your observations and record them after the treatment. A record of your efforts will help ensure that you remember all the details from one massage to another and therefore appreciate the progress made, especially if you have several dogs to massage. Think of your dog as a very picky, demanding client who is always checking on you. You want to give him the best massage possible.

Your Dog's Feedback Signs

Part of your "dog sense" is to be aware of the feedback signs the dog gives you. Learn to recognize the sure signs of apprehension: raising or turning the head towards you, eyes widening and becoming intense, skin twitching or flinching, fidgeting, tensing up, moving away from the pressure, breathing short and hard, whimpering or short to long yelping sounds.

On the other hand, eyes half closed, head down, ears to the side, heavy sighs are sure signs of relaxation and enjoyment. Monitor your dog's body language constantly and adjust your work accordingly.

Pain and discomfort feedback signs from your dog should always be regarded as a warning signal, therefore pay attention! Sudden jolts or tensing during the massage can indicate that the pressure you are applying is too strong, or you have found a significant tender spot, or that simply your dog is afraid of what you are doing. Take time to reassure your dog with a soft voice and gentle rubbing.

Owing to his genetic inheritance, certain parts of the dog's body have special social or psychological associations. For example, when you start massaging your dog, he may roll on his back right away, presenting you his abdomen as a sign of submission and willingness to be massaged. Female dogs when in heat may raise their hind end and present it sexually when you start massaging the base of the tail. For the male dog, the

A

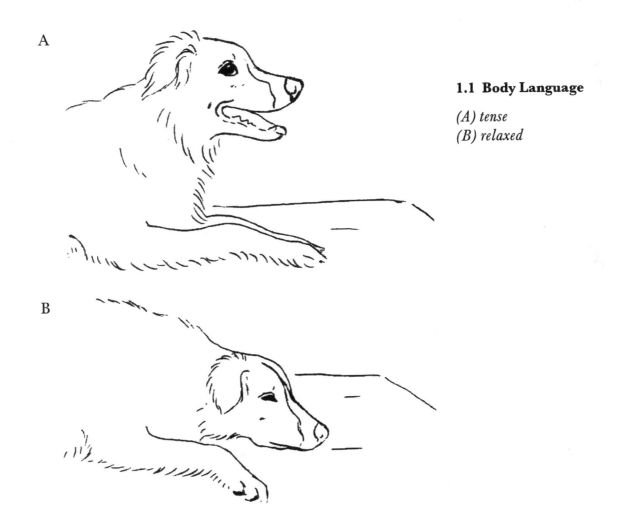

B

1.1 Body Language

(A) tense
(B) relaxed

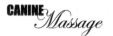

groin or inguinal area is a very important body region. A dog presents his groin for contact as a sign of friendship or a submissive gesture to other dogs and people alike.

The neck area, the "scruff of the neck," is often a "shy spot" because of the grabbing and biting that is associated with dominance and fighting. Some male dogs may be agitated when you start working the neck area.

Also remember that intense restlessness, even 10 minutes into the massage, may indicate that the dog has a strong need to urinate. To avoid accidents, make sure to take your dog out before the massage.

The Dog's Response

Like humans, most dogs enjoy massage therapy when it is done with skilled hands. During their first massage experience, most dogs are very curious about what is happening to them and some may even display a defensive attitude. If he feels nervous or impatient, often a dog will move away. If this happens, do not hesitate to use firm commands to calm him, and when he obeys, praise him. Try to make this first experience fun and use lots of praise. Be patient about the results as well as with your dog.

Because dogs are social animals who strive to please their owners, they often respond well to a positive, reassuring voice using lots of praise. Always talk to your dog in a quiet, peaceful way when starting a massage. It will work well to settle him down, especially during the first massage.

After a few sessions, most dogs will accept massage without any trouble and will enjoy it. Unfortunately some dogs, due to improper handling, lack of training and/or bonding with humans during their early years or traumatic histories of accidents or abuse, may be more fearful of massage. They experience what I call "touch-shyness", which cause them to tense up all over. Time, patience, love and massage care will do wonders for this type of animal. Regular massage sessions, even if short, will definitely help this type of animal ease their fears. They learn to trust, resulting in better behavior and handling.

When dealing with an extreme case of phobia or restlessness, have your veterinarian check the dog. A mild tranquilizer for the first few massage sessions might be in order. In some cases, "touch-shyness" in particular areas of the body (head, neck, paws or back) can indicate an underlying condition or sickness. Make sure that you check with your veterinarian before proceeding with the massage.

Take the time to study the dog's temperament and character to make the proper connection during the first massage. Most dogs and puppies respond very positively to their first treatment. Puppies may engage in playful fighting with your hands during the massage. I recommend that when dealing with a young dog, massage him after a good exercise workout or play workout so he will be tired and ready for some quiet massage time.

As a rule, use the relaxation routine from Chapter 7 prior to giving any massage, at any time, and to any dog. Don't rush! With each session you will build your dog's trust while allaying his instinctive fears. As the dog relaxes during the session, his head will go down and its breathing will become deeper and slower with occasional sighing. To encourage the dog, praise him a lot when this occurs. Sighing is a definite indication of tension release. You will feel a strong energy field around the animal as he relaxes. Depending on the nature of the massage you use, the dog may either go to sleep or may perk up and be ready for exercise. Some dogs, like people, prefer a deeper and heavier massage, while others prefer a lighter and softer massage. You will be able to cue in on your animal's tolerance by starting slowly and gently to first trigger a relaxation response. Then, by gradually increasing your pressure and depth of work, you will be able to reach deep into the muscular and connective tissues without causing your dog to tense up or to try to get away from you. Indeed, if you use too heavy a pressure or manipulate the muscular tissue too hastily, your dog will let you know by tensing up or even yelping. Adjust your work accordingly and reassure your dog with lots of soft spoken feedback.

Positioning the Dog

When working on an average or large size dog, it is recommended you use a sturdy table with a comfortable blanket or large cushion on it. The proper height for this "massage table" should be measured in relation to your height. The measurement from the floor to your wrist should be equal to the height of the table with the pillow on it. A table at the correct height will help you to maintain good posture—back straight, shoulder and arms relaxed—and avoid fatigue and muscle tension. A table that is either too high or too low will cause back and shoulder muscle tension to develop. To make the table accessible for your dog, use some kind of stairway, like a stool, a chair or a plastic crate for it to climb up on.

When working on a small size dog, you can sit comfortably with your back straight, and have a large pillow on your lap for your dog to lie on. Keep your back straight and arms relaxed.

It is not recommended you give a massage to your dog while on the floor with you kneeling and bending over. This position will cause you lots of unnecessary discomfort and eventually pain, while in turn rendering your massage less efficient than if you were properly positioned and relaxed.

1.2 Correct Table Height

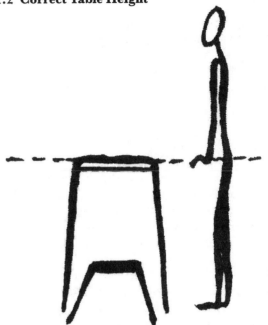

Duration of a Massage

Your first massage - and especially if it is the animal's first massage - should last between 5 and 8 minutes. Use your own judgment in relation to the dog's size, temperament and feedback signs. The very first massage is a very special moment in which you should really emphasize a soft, mindful and caring contact to gain the animal's trust.

For the first full body massage, again proceed gently and in a very relaxed manner, avoiding hasty rhythm and deep pressure, until the dog

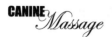

has become confident in your work. This massage should last between 15 and 20 minutes, up to 30 minutes for large dogs. After several sessions you can increase the time frame of your massages to 30 minutes. It is not unusual to spend 45 minutes on a thorough maintenance routine with a large dog accustomed to massage.

A maintenance massage routine (see Chapter 7) can be done at any time to keep the animal's muscular structure fit; it should last 15 or 20 minutes in the early practice and up to 30 minutes, depending on the dog's size. A recuperation routine should be used after the dog has exercised so as to prevent stiffness or tying-up; it should run between 10 and 15 minutes.

The dog's temperament plays an important role in its receptivity to massage. Most dogs will become restless, almost agitated, after a 30 minute massage, but some animals can easily take over 30 minutes of a gentle, in-depth maintenance massage.

Your connection with the dog is important. When massaging a "stranger" for the first time, do not expect too much. But after several massage sessions, most dogs will love being massaged; they will lower their heads and go into relaxation mode very quickly. That's their way of showing you that they appreciate your work!

When working on a specific area, for example a large area such as the hind quarters or the back, you should not spend more than 5 to 10 minutes on that part, otherwise you risk overworking the structures. Such overwork could result in inflammation and irritation of the tissues. For the same reason, do not spend more than 5 minutes on a small area such as the upper neck or the stifle.

Judge the situation carefully. Consider the state of the tissues and the dog's tolerance at the time of treatment.

Evaluate and plan your massage mentally before you start, keeping track of time as you move around the body. With practice, this technique will become second nature to you.

When to Massage Your Dog

Depending on your goals and the situation at hand, you need to find the most suitable time in order to achieve the best results. Basically, any time is a good time to massage your dog, but you want to choose the moment when your dog will be most receptive.

The most effective use of massage therapy is to integrate the massage into your everyday routine of working with your animal. For example, you can massage right after grooming, after exercise, or when putting your dog away for the night. You can choose a morning or evening schedule for a thorough, full-body session. You are the judge and common sense is the rule. In any case, always observe the following guidelines:

- Always perform a "health" check to ensure that there are no contra-indications prevailing prior to massaging the animal.

- Develop a routine and base your work on it. A repetitive pattern ensures confidence and relaxation.

When you want to deliver a good massage to your animal, it is best to wait for the dog's "moment". Evaluating your dog's temperament will help you discover its "best time." If yours is a "morning dog", work in the morning. If an "afternoon dog", work in the afternoon. If a "night dog," work in the late evening. Once your dog has experienced the "magic" of your hands, it will often come up to you, and lean against you to "beg" for a rub, moving around so that you massage just where he wants you to.

The training and lifestyle your dog is used to will also play a role in determining a good time for a massage. Here are a few examples of different massage routines and a dog's activity: a maintenance massage before exercise; a recuperation routine after exercise; a relaxation massage before bed time, after a long day, before and after traveling, when restless or in pain. Also, keep in mind outside influences that can affect your dog: abnormal activities going on in the house, construction, visitors, arrival of a new dog or other pet, an approaching electrical storm, strong winds, and so on. A dog may also be restless because of extremely hot weather, a heavy training schedule with very rich food, and during competition, traveling, and feeding time.

Remember, a relaxation routine (see Chapter 7 for more on the variety of massage routines) can be done at any time. It is always used to start a full body massage. The relaxation routine works wonders in switching a dog's mood, especially if it is depressed, naughty, mischievous or simply tense.

A maintenance routine is best done when the dog is warm, after some exercise either morning or evening. If the dog cannot be warmed by exercises, cover it with a blanket or use hot water bottle to increase circulation.

The warm up routine is always done before heavy training or a play workout. This routine helps the dog warm up its muscle structure and prevent possible muscle tear.

The recuperation routine is always done after heavy playing or training. This routine helps the dog recover faster by eliminating toxins in a matter of a few hours.

Massage after injury should be worked into a schedule followed by stretching exercises, or a rest period, depending on the recovery development. Remember to work with your veterinarian to ensure maximum benefit to your dog.

Do's and Don'ts

The ambiance in which you work will directly influence the efficiency of the massage. Here are some guidelines for you to observe in order to ensure maximum safety for both you and the dog when giving a massage.

Do's:

✓ Do check with your veterinarian if you suspect your dog is not feeling well. Ensure there are no contra-indications prevailing.

✓ Do maintain a soothing atmosphere: not too much traffic, not too many noises. Eventually you may play peaceful, quiet music.

✓ Do keep other pets away.

✓ Do work indoors.

✓ Do use a massage table cushioned with a blanket or large pillow. Keep the area around the table free of obstacles.

✓ Do allow the dog complete freedom of head movement since this allows for better relaxation and for more feed-back signals to you.

✓ Do wait after strenuous exercise.

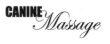

✓ Do wait two hours after eating.

✓ Do check your dog and remove burrs, mud, etc. before you begin a massage.

✓ Do always start massaging with a very light pressure and progress to deeper work.

✓ Do keep your fingernails short and avoid wearing jewelry and heavy perfume.

✓ Do keep talking to the animal throughout the massage session.

✓ Do always pay attention to the feedback signs (eyes, ears, tail, breathing, noise and changes in posture).

✓ Do keep records of your observations and the types of massage you give.

✓ Do establish a massage and exercise schedule for the following weeks or until recovery if the dog is injured.

✓ Do wear loose fitting clothing to give yourself freedom of movement.

Don'ts:

✗ Don't disregard the physiological signs of contra-indications.

✗ Don't allow loud music, commotion, smoking.

✗ Don't allow other pets to wander around. Prevent such an intrusion before starting the massage session.

✗ Don't work in a narrow space.

✗ Don't work on a dirty dog—one with mud or burrs on his body.

✗ Don't work hastily, too quickly or too forcefully.

✗ Don't have long fingernails or wear jewelry.

✗ Don't stop verbal feed-back to the dog; he needs praise and reassurance.

✗ Don't talk loudly or shout.

✗ Don't talk to somebody else while working. You will lose your concentration and this will affect the quality of your work. The dog will definitely feel the difference.

✗ Don't use heavy pressure at the start.

✗ Don't ignore feedback signs from the dog (eyes, ears, tail, breathing, noise).

✗ Don't work right after heavy exercise or eating.

✗ Don't be angry or in a bad mood when working on a dog.

✗ Don't think negatively.

Contra-indications to Massaging a Dog

Contra-indications refer to the specific situations in which you should not massage a dog. If these conditions exist, consult your veterinarian first. For example:

✗ Do not massage a dog with a temperature over 104° F or 39.5° C. A dog's regular temperature is 101° F or 38.5° C. An increase in temperature occurs during serious illness— usually an ill dog is depressed, off his feed and doesn't want to move. Feverish conditions necessitate complete rest. Massage will only worsen the situation by increasing an already accelerated blood circulation. Check with your vet. The laying on of hands over the head and over the sacrum area will soothe the dog.

✗ When your dog is suffering from shock.

✗ When there is an open (broken skin) or healing (bleeding) wound, avoid that particular area. You may massage the rest of the body to release compensatory tension or excess swelling.

✗ When there is acute trauma such as a torn muscle or an area with internal bleeding such as an acute hematoma following a strong blow. Have a veterinarian evaluate this condition immediately. Use ice for the first few hours. Massage can resume in the chronic stage, usually after 72 hours.

✗ When there is an acute sprain, use ice until the initial swelling goes down, then use the swelling technique from Chapter 6.

✗ When there are severe forms of functional nervous diseases such as acute disc disease, for example, the nerve stimulation would make the dog extremely uncomfortable.

✗ Acute nerve problems or nerve irritation (neuralgia) in a particular area following a wound or a bad stretch. The laying on of hands may soothe. Use cold hydrotherapy to numb the nerve endings before and after the laying on of hands.

✗ During colitis, diarrhea, pregnancy or hernias, use just a light stroking on the abdomen and only if the dog does not mind.

✗ Acute arthritis can be too painful to permit massage. Massage could worsen the inflammation. Instead, use cold hydrotherapy locally. Once the acute stage is relieved, resume your massage. Chronic stages of rheumatism and arthritis require a different massage treatment. Light massage over the areas affected will relax the compensatory tension from the muscles supporting those structures. Do not work deeply around the joints.

✗ Inflammatory conditions such as phlebitis would be worsened by direct massage. Use cold hydrotherapy and check with your veterinarian.

✗ Tumors and cysts of cancerous origin are contra-indicated; massage will spread them. Avoid the affected areas but you may massage the rest of the body. Check with your vet

Massage is formally contra-indicated in the following conditions, since massage may spread the problem:

✗ Skin problems of fungal origin such as ringworm and bacterial skin disease.

✗ Acute stages of any infectious diseases.

Be careful when dealing with what appears to be an abnormal situation. When in doubt, contact a veterinarian. When massage is contra-indicated, it is best to keep your dog warm, properly hydrated and undisturbed. Follow

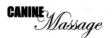
CANINE *Massage*

your veterinarian's advice with medication. The laying of hands will often soothe an irritated area (see Chapter 5). Hydrotherapy, discussed later, also will relieve the inflammation and pain considerably, assisting recovery and definitively comforting your animal.

Knowing how to safely approach an animal for massage is part of the secret to a successful massage. Your patience, perseverance, good humor, kindness, knowledge and skills will reduce the psychological and physical barrier between the dog and you, leading to better communication with the animal.

General Anatomy and Physiology of the Dog

CHAPTER 2

Knowing some of the anatomy and physiology of your dog will help you develop a better ability to "feel-see" when massaging your pet, as well as sharpening your massage skills. In this chapter, information will be provided about the various systems that make up the anatomy of the dog. Detailed information concerning each individual system is beyond the scope of this book, however since massage mostly deals with the musculoskeletal system which induces body movement, I will describe the nervous system, the skeletal system, and the muscular system in greater detail to further your understanding.

The nine principal systems of the body are:

1. Nervous
2. Skeletal
3. Muscular
4. Circulatory
5. Respiratory
6. Digestive
7. Urinary
8. Endocrine
9. Reproductive

The dog's health depends on the harmonious working relationship of all these body systems.

The Nervous System

The nervous system (the brain, spinal cord, sensory and motor nerves) controls the workings of all other systems. The nervous system integrates and controls every body function, both voluntary and involuntary; it processes all information and governs all commands to the body. Within the nervous system are found:

- The central nervous system. The CNS is made up of the brain and spinal cord, which perform very specific functions. Massage does not directly affect the CNS, only indirectly via the peripheral nervous system (PNS).

- The peripheral nervous system. The PNS conveys nerve impulses through the efferent or motor nerves that carry information from the CNS to the body parts, and the afferent or sensory nerves that carry information from the body parts to the CNS. These nerves exit the spinal column at the vertebrae. Massage

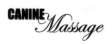

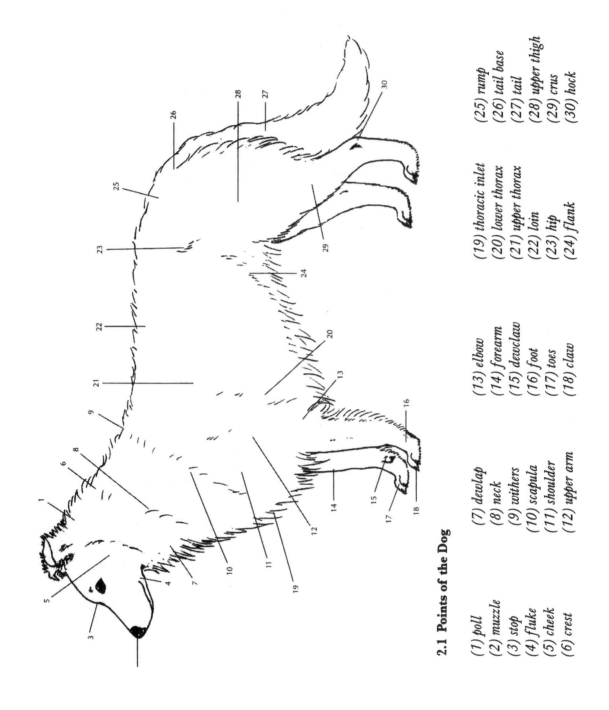

2.1 Points of the Dog

(1) poll
(2) muzzle
(3) stop
(4) fluke
(5) cheek
(6) crest

(7) dewlap
(8) neck
(9) withers
(10) scapula
(11) shoulder
(12) upper arm

(13) elbow
(14) forearm
(15) dewclaw
(16) foot
(17) toes
(18) claw

(19) thoracic inlet
(20) lower thorax
(21) upper thorax
(22) loin
(23) hip
(24) flank

(25) rump
(26) tail base
(27) tail
(28) upper thigh
(29) crus
(30) hock

directly influences the PNS via pressure and rhythm.

The PNS's nerve tissues are composed of many filaments that are very susceptible to pressure. In the case of a strong trauma, when significant or severe pressure is applied to a nerve, nerve impulses can stop traveling along it. As a consequence, two things can happen: the loss of sensation or feedback due to the loss of sensory nerve impulses from a body part to the CNS and the degeneration and eventual shrinking of the tissue in the immediate area of the affected nerve as a result of lost motor nerve impulses from the CNS to the body part.

The overall functioning of the nervous system is ensured by the Autonomic Nervous System (ANS), which maintains a stable internal environment. The ANS governs the vital organs and their complex functions that are normally carried out involuntarily, such as breathing, circulation, digestion, elimination and the immune response. The ANS also helps coordinate the locomotor function for safety and smoothness of movements of the body during action.

The Autonomic Nervous System has two major divisions: the sympathetic and the parasympathetic. Both originate in the brain.

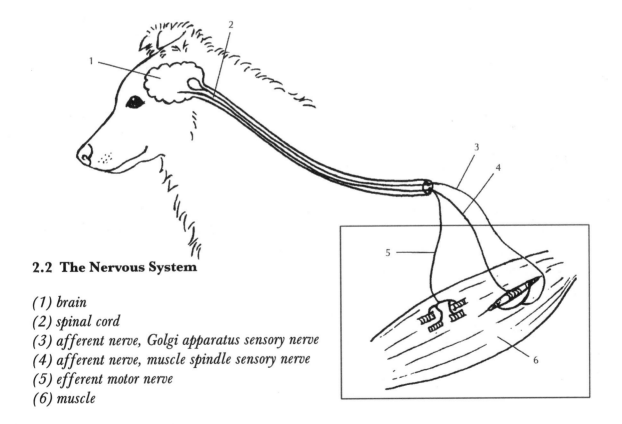

2.2 The Nervous System

(1) brain
(2) spinal cord
(3) afferent nerve, Golgi apparatus sensory nerve
(4) afferent nerve, muscle spindle sensory nerve
(5) efferent motor nerve
(6) muscle

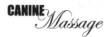

The sympathetic division causes the body to respond to danger, adversity, stress, anger and ecstasy by increasing the heart rate, blood pressure, the volume of air exchange and the volume of blood flowing to the muscles - all of which are needed for the dog to spring into action. The sympathetic division is often described as the "fight or flight" division. Many massage routines or techniques will cause a general stimulation of the sympathetic division resulting in mobilization of resources to prepare the body to act or to deal with emergencies.

The parasympathetic division monitors body functions during times of sickness, rest, sleep, digestion and elimination when the body is not ready to spring into action. A general stimulation of the parasympathetic promotes relaxation and the vegetative functions of the body such as breathing, circulation, digestion, immune response and reproduction. The "relaxation routine" discussed later is designed to relax the nervous system.

The Skeletal System

The skeletal system serves as a framework for the dog's body, giving the muscles something to work against and defining the animal's overall size and shape. The skeleton also protects the dog's vital internal tissues and organs: for example, the skull protects the brain; the rib cage protects the lungs and heart; the vertebral column protects the spinal cord.

Bones

Bones come in different shapes and sizes and have specific functions. With the exception of the teeth, which are enamel-covered, bones are the body's hardest tissues. They are made up of min-eral, mostly calcium. Bones are capable of withstanding great compression, torque, and tension. The periosteum, a tough connective tissue membrane, covers and protects each bone. It provides for the attachment of the joint capsules, the ligaments and the tendons. Injury to the periosteum may result in undesirable bone growths. Bones are held together by ligaments; muscles are attached to the bones by tendons. The articulating surface of the bone is covered with a thick, smooth cartilage that diminishes concussion and friction.

There are long bones in the limbs; short bones in the wrist, knee and hock; flat bones in the rib cage, skull and shoulder blade; and irregular bones in the vertebrae of the spinal column, sacrum, and tail, as well as some bones of the skull.

Long bones function mainly as levers and aid in the support of weight. For example, the foreleg includes the humerus, radius, ulna bones, and the hind leg includes the femur and tibia and fibula bones.

Short bones, such as the carpus (wrist) and tarsus (hock) are found in complex joints and absorb concussion.

The flat bones protect and enclose the cavities containing vital organs. They also provide large areas for the attachment of muscles, for example, the shoulder blades and hips. Both long and flat bones have a central cavity that produces special cells, including bone marrow.

So-called irregular bones have many bony projections of various shapes and sizes that offer attachments for muscles, tendons and ligaments. For example, vertebrae are irregular bones in the spi-

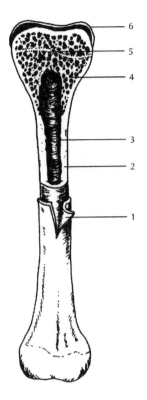

2.3 Parts of a Bone

(1) periosteum
(2) compact bone
(3) medullary cavity
(4) spongy bone with marrow cavities
(5) epiphyseal plate
(6) articulate hyaline cartilage

nal column that provide solid anchoring for loco-motor muscle groups.

The skeleton is made up of:

- The skull and its facial bones - nasal, frontal, parietal and jaw bones;

- The spine, with its 7 cervical, 13 thoracic, 7 lumbar and 3 fused sacral vertebrae. The tail is usually made up of 20 to 23 caudal vertebrae, although this number can vary considerably;

- The rib cage, made up of 13 pairs of ribs springing from the thoracic vertebrae, curving forward and downward, meeting at the sternum (breastbone);

- The forelegs, which carry 60 percent of the dog's body weight. The thoracic limb is comprised of the scapula (shoulder blade), the humerus, the radius and ulna, carpus bones, the metacarpus and phalanges.

The hind legs (or pelvic limb) is comprised of the pelvis (ilium, ischium and pubis); the femur, the tibia and fibula; the hock or tarsus which includes seven tarsal bones, the metatarsals and phalanges.

Joints

The joints permit certain parts of the bony frame to articulate and produce motion. Joints are the meeting places between two bones. Movement

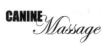

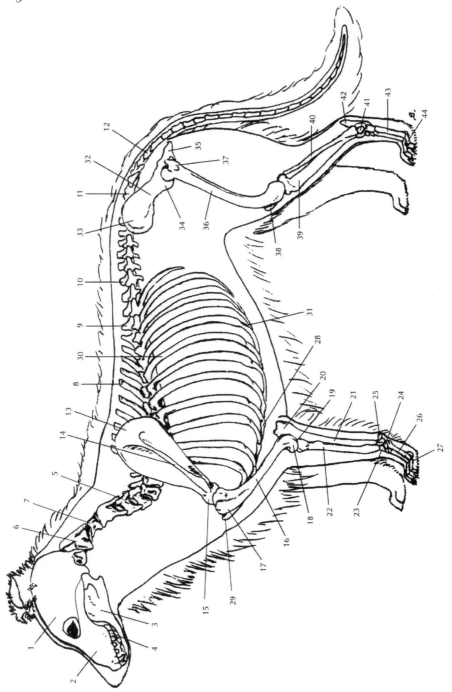

2.4 Skeleton of the Dog

(1) cranium
(2) maxilla
(3) mandible
(4) teeth
(5) cervical vertebrae - 7
(6) atlas (first cervical vertebra)
(7) axis (second vervical vertebra)
(8) thoracic vertebrae - 13
(9) last thoracic vertebra
(10) lumbar vertebrae - 7
(11) sacrum (3 fused vertebrae)
(12) caudal vertebrae (usually 18)
(13) scapula
(14) scapular spine
(15) neck of scapula
(16) humerus
(17) greater tubercle
(18) lateral condyle of humerus
(19) elbow joint
(20) olecranon process of the unla
(21) unla
(22) radius

(23) carpus
(24) carpal bones
(25) pisiforme bone
(26) metacarpal bones
(27) phalanges
(28) sternum (breastbone)
(29) manubrium sternum
(30) rib
(31) costal cartilage
(32) pelvis
(33) ilium
(34) pubis
(35) ischium
(36) femur
(37) greater trochanter
(38) patella
(39) tibia
(40) fibula
(41) tarsal bones
(42) tuber calcanei
(43) metatarsus
(44) phalanges

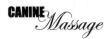
of the dog is dependent upon the contraction of muscles and the corresponding articulation of the joints.

Some joints are not movable and are referred to as fibrous or cartilaginous joints because they lack a joint cavity. Immovable joints include the sacro-iliac, the bones forming the pelvis, and the skull.

But most joints in the body are movable. They are called synovial joints and include the shoulder, elbow, carpus, stifle and hock, all of which permit a great range of motion. The ends of the bones are lined with hyaline cartilage which pro-vides a smooth surface between the bones and acts as a shock-absorber during times of compression, such as when jumping or during quick turns. Joints are also surrounded by joint capsules, also known as the capsular ligaments. The inner layer of the capsular wall is made up of a delicate layer of synovial membrane, which produces a viscous, lubricating secretion known as the synovial fluid.

A joint can perform many movements, including flexion (bending), extension, abduction (drawing away from the middle of the body), adduction (drawing back to the center), and rotation.

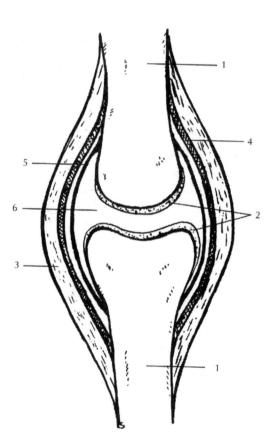

2.5 Parts of a Joint

(1) bone
(2) hyaline cartilage
(3) ligament
(4) fibrous capsule
(5) synovial lining
(6) joint cavity (with synovial fluid)

Ligaments

A ligament is a band of connective tissue that links one bone to another. Tendons connect muscles to bones. Ligaments are made up of collagen, a fibrous protein found in the connective tissue. Ligaments have a limited blood supply and because of this injuries or sprains take longer than in a muscle.

Most ligaments are located around joints to give extra support, to prevent an excessive or abnormal range of motion and to resist the pressure of lateral torque (a twisting motion).

Ligaments are very tough. Ligaments have very little contraction power. Therefore they must work in conjunction with muscles. Within very narrow limits, ligaments are somewhat elastic. From human sport medicine we know that if a ligament is overstretched or repeatedly stretched, it might lose up to 25 percent of its strength; such a ligament may need surgical repair to recover its full tensile strength. Severe ligament sprain will lead to joint instability.

Several ligamentous structures help support and protect the vertebral column, pelvis, neck and limbs from suddenly imposed strain.

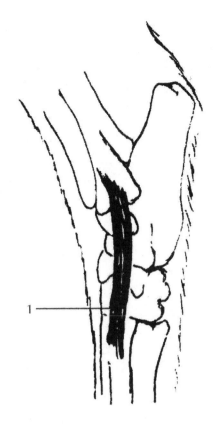

2.6 A Ligament

(1) Lateral collateral ligament of tarsal joint

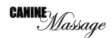

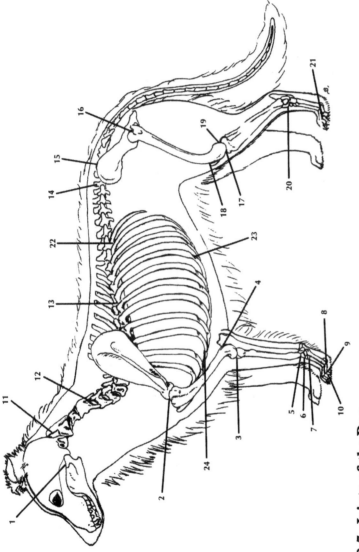

2.7 Joints of the Dog

(1) temporomandibular (tmj)
(2) shoulder
(3) elbow, humeroradial component
(4) elbow, humeroulnar component
(5) carpus, radiocarpal
(6) carpus, intercarpal
(7) carpometacarpal
(8) metacarpophalangeal
(9) proximal interphalangeal
(10) distal interphalangeal
(11) atlantoccipital
(12) cervical intervertebral
(13) thoracic intervertebral
(14) lumbosacral
(15) sacroiliac
(16) hip
(17) stifle
(18) femoropatellar component of stifle
(19) femorotibial component of stifle
(20) tarsus (hock)
(21) metatarsophalangeal
(22) costovertebral
(23) costochondral
(24) costosternal

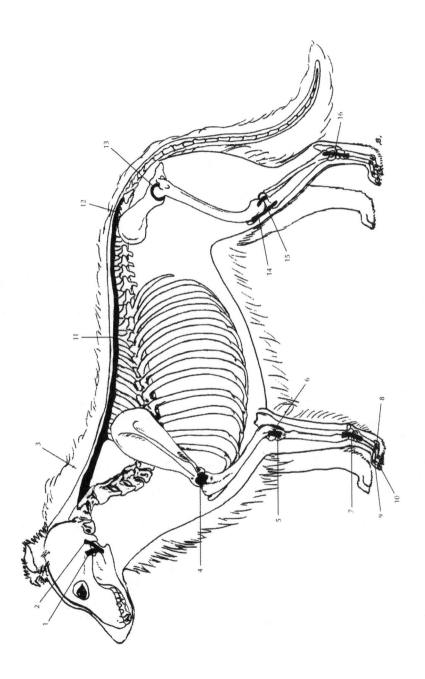

2.8 Representative Ligaments of the Dog as Seen Laterally

(1) lateral ligaments of temporomandibular joint
(2) caudal ligaments of the temporomandibular joint
(3) nuchal ligament
(4) capsular ligament of shoulder joint
(5) lateral collateral ligament of elbow joint
(6) annular radioulnar ligament
(7) lateral collateral ligament of carpal joint
(8) lateral collateral ligament of metacarpophalangeal joint

(9) collateral ligament of proximal interphalangeal joint
(10) collateral ligament of distal interphalangeal joint
(11) supraspinous ligament
(12) supraspinous ligament (sacral portion)
(13) capsular ligament of hip joint
(14) patellar ligament
(15) lateral collateral ligament of stifle joint
(16) lateral collateral ligament of tarsal joint

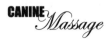

2.9 Cross-Section of a Skeletal Muscle

(1) tendon
(2) muscle belly
(3) muscle fiber (containing thick and thin filaments)
(4) bundles (made up of fibers)
(5) fascia

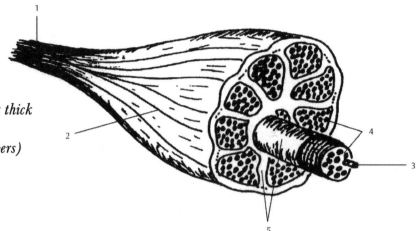

The Muscular System

The muscular system provides the power and means to move the bony frame. There are three classes of muscle: smooth, cardiac and skeletal. The smooth and cardiac muscles are involuntary, or autonomic; they play a part in the digestive, respiratory, circulatory and urogenital systems. For the most part, the skeletal muscle is voluntary; it functions in the dog's movements. In massage, we are concerned with the more than 700 skeletal muscles that are responsible for movement in the dog.

There are at least two main types of muscle fiber: slow twitch fibers (ST) and fast twitch fibers (FT).

• ST fibers are aerobic fibers and need oxygen to do their job. Thus ST fibers require a good supply of blood to bring oxygen to them and to remove waste products created during exercise. ST fibers also have strong endurance qualities.

• FT fibers are anaerobic fibers; they do not need oxygen to work and therefore are able to deliver the quick muscular effort required for a sudden burst of speed. However, FT fibers are only able to perform for short periods of time.

The ratio of ST to FT fibers is genetically inherited. Careful selective breeding can emphasize these features in a dog.

Regardless of the FT/ST fibers ratio, a muscle is made up of a fleshy part and two tendon attachments. The muscle belly, or fleshy part, is the part that contracts in response to a nervous command. During contraction, the muscle fibers basically fold on themselves, which shortens them and results in muscle movement. The muscle belly is made up of many muscle fibers arranged in bundles with each bundle wrapped in connective tissue (fascia). The fascia covers, supports and separates each individual muscle bundle and the whole muscle itself. This arrangement allows for greater support, strength and flexibility in the movement between each of the muscle groups.

Tendons

A tendon is the muscle part that attaches to the bone. Tendons are made up of connective tissue — a dense, white fibrous tissue much like that of a ligament. The tendon of origin is the tendon that attaches the muscle to the less-movable bone, whereas the tendon of insertion is the tendon that attaches the muscle to the more-movable bone, so that on contraction the insertion is brought closer to the origin. Tendons attach to the periosteum of the bone; the fibers of the tendon blend with the periosteum fibers because of their similar collagen make-up. Tendons can be fairly short or quite long as seen on some of the flexor and extensor muscles of the lower legs. Usually, tendons are rounded but they can be flattened like the tendons attached along the spine or like the aponeurosis tendon of the external abdominal oblique muscle.

Because of their high-tensile strength, tendons can endure an enormous amount of tension, usually more than the muscle itself can produce; conse-

quently, tendons do not rupture easily. They are not as elastic as muscle fibers, but they are more elastic than ligament fibers.

Tendons can "stress up" after heavy exercise, meaning that they can stay contracted. Gentle massage and stretching will loosen residual tension.

Inflamed tendons are at great risk of being strained or overstretched. Many leg muscles have long tendons that run down the leg over the joints. These tendons are protected by sheaths or "tendon bursa". Chronic irritation of the sheath can result in excess fluid production and soft swellings. Stirring up the blood circulation with massage and cold hydrotherapy will help circulation and keep inflammation down. If the inflammation persists, check with your veterinarian.

Skeletal Muscles

Muscles come in all shapes and sizes. Some are small and some large, some are thin and some are bulky. Look at the muscle charts to note the variety of shapes in the dog's muscle structure.

Muscles act together to give the dog its grace and power. Muscles work in three different ways: isometric contraction, concentric contrac-

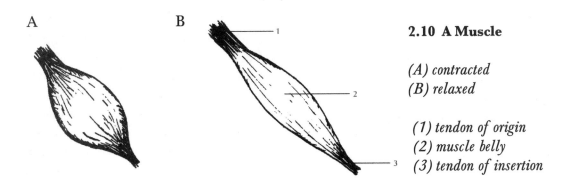

A   B

2.10 A Muscle

(A) contracted
(B) relaxed

(1) tendon of origin
(2) muscle belly
(3) tendon of insertion

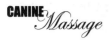

tion and eccentric contraction. Isometric contraction occurs when a muscle contracts without causing any movement. During standing, for example, isometric contraction ensures stability. Concentric contraction occurs when a muscle shortens as it contracts causing articular movements. Concentric contraction is mostly seen in regular movements such as protraction (forward movement) or retraction (backward movement) of the limbs and in any movement of the neck or back. Eccentric contraction occurs when a muscle gradually releases as it elongates. Eccentric contraction assists regular movements by avoiding jerky unstable actions; it also plays a role in shock absorption during the landing phase of jumping.

Skeletal muscles are highly elastic and have strong contractile power. They respond to motor nerve impulses and as a result, the contraction mechanism is a generated process. The release process is not a generated process but, rather, it is a natural relaxation of the muscle as a result of the cessation of the motor nerve impulses that originally asked the muscle to contract.

Muscles are equipped with two types of sensory nerve endings: the Golgi apparatus and the muscle spindle.

The Golgi apparatus nerve endings send feedback impulses to the brain as to the whereabouts of the muscle; this process is referred to as proprioception. The Golgi nerve endings are mostly located where the muscle and the tendons come together.

The muscle spindle nerve endings prevent overstretching of the muscle fibers. As its name implies, this nerve fiber coils around the length of the muscle bundle. When reaching a given length, the muscle spindle fires nerve impulses that trigger a fast reflex motor nerve reaction to induce immediate contraction of the muscle fibers. Thus the overstretching and potential tearing of fibers is prevented. This is a safety reflex mechanism.

When a muscle develops a contracture, the muscle fibers stay contracted. This could result in a spasm. With a contracture the natural relaxation process will not happen but pain and motion problems (restriction) will.

When a muscle overstretches, a spasm often results. A spasm is a violent contraction of a muscle in response to overstretching or trauma whereby the muscle is unable to release its rigidity. A microspasm, or stress point, however, is a small spasm occurring in just a few fibers of the muscle bundle. Microspasms have a cumulative effect over a period of time resulting in a full spasm.

Sometimes a muscle is stretched past its limits and muscle fibers will tear. This causes an immediate muscle spasm and triggers an inflammation response with swelling at the site of injury. As part of the healing process, new connective tissue is laid down in an irregular scattered pattern within the muscle fiber arrangement. Unfortunately this scar tissue reduces the muscle tensile strength, flexibility and elasticity. Massage therapy can reduce the amount of scar tissue by applying kneading and friction after proper warm up of the tissues. Also, stretching is a great technique to prevent and reduce the formation of scar tissue.

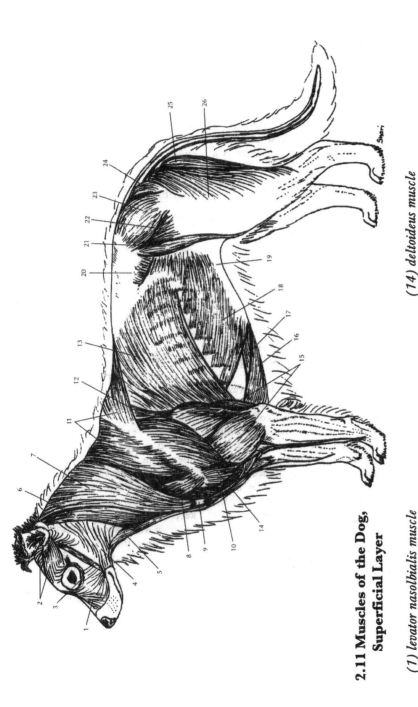

2.11 Muscles of the Dog, Superficial Layer

(1) levator nasolbialis muscle
(2) frontalis
(3) orbicularis oculi
(4) cervical subcutaneous muscle
(5) sternohyoideus muscle
(6) sternocephalicus muscle
(7) brachiocephalicus muscle, par cervicalis
(8) omotransversarius muscle
(9) clavicular band
(10) cleidobrachialis muscle
(11) trapezius cervicus and thoracis muscle
(12) infraspinatus muscle
(13) latissimus dorsi muscle

(14) deltoideus muscle
(15) triceps brachii muscle (long and lateral head)
(16) deep pectoral muscle
(17) rectus abdominus muscle
(18) external abdominal oblique muscle
(19) aponeurosis
(20) lumbar fascia
(21) sartorius muscle
(22) tensor fascia latae muscle
(23) middle gluteal muscle
(24) superficial gluteal muscle
(25) semitendinosus muscle
(26) biceps femoris muscle

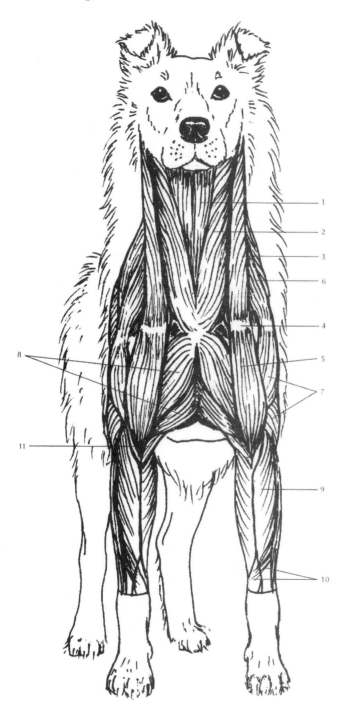

**2.12 Muscles of the Dog,
Anterior (Front) View**

(1)   sternohyoideus muscle
(2)   sternomastoideus muscle
(3)   brachiocephalicus muscle, par cervicalis
(4)   clavicular band
(5)   cleidobrachialis muscle
(6)   omotransversarius muscle
(7)   triceps muscle, long & lateral head
(8)   pectoralis major superficialis muscle
(9)   extensor carpi radialis muscle
(10) abductor pollicis longus muscle
(11) biceps brachii muscle

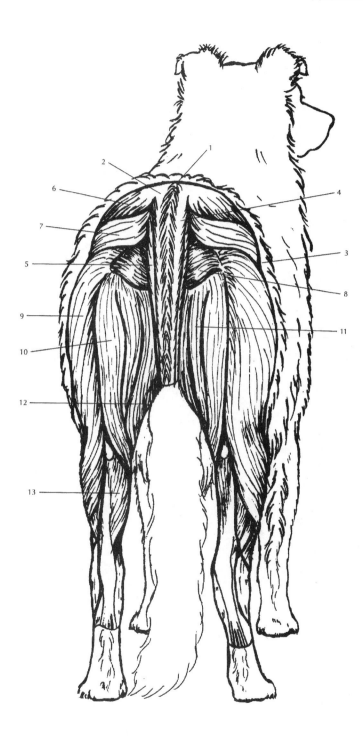

2.13 Muscles of the Dog, Posterior (Rear) View

(1) lumbar fascia
(2) dock of the tail
(3) point of hip or haunch
      (tuber coxae)
(4) levator muscles of tail
(5) depressor muscles of tail
(6) middle gluteal muscle
(7) superficial gluteal muscle
(8) ischiatic tuberosity
(9) biceps femoris muscle
(10) semitendinosus muscle
(11) semimembranosus muscle
(12) gracilis muscle
(13) gastrocnemius muscle

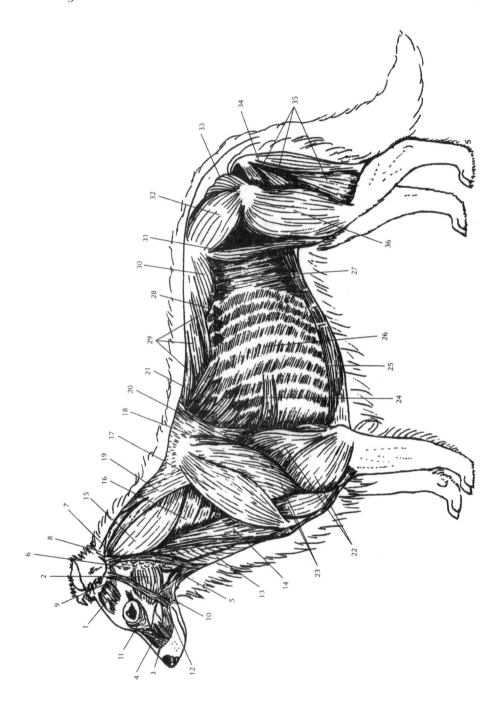

2.14 Muscles of the Dog, Deeper Layer

(1) temporalis muscle
(2) masseter muscle
(3) nasolabialis muscle
(4) buccalis muscle
(5) parotid salivary gland
(6) submandibular salivary gland
(7) parotidoauricular muscle
(8) occipitalis muscle
(9) zygomaticoauricularis muscle
(10) digastricus muscle
(11) orbicularis oculi muscle
(12) orbicularis oris muscle
(13) sternomastoideus muscle
(14) brachiocephalicus muscle
(15) splenius muscle
(16) serratus ventralis cervicis muscle
(17) supraspinatus muscle
(18) infraspinatus muscle

(19) rhomboideus muscle
(20) teres major muscle
(21) serratus dorsalis thoracis muscle
(22) triceps brachii muscle, long & lateral head
(23) deltoideus muscle
(24) scalenus muscle
(25) rectus abdominus muscle
(26) intercostal muscle
(27) transversus abdominus muscle
(28) serratus dorsalis caudalis muscle
(29) longissimus dorsi muscle
(30) iliocostalis muscle
(31) satorius muscle
(32) middle gluteal muscle
(33) superficial gluteal muscle
(34) semimembranosus muscle
(35) semitendinosus muscle
(36) quadriceps femoris muscle

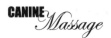

A heavily exercised muscle will often develop a light inflammation within its fibers. This is a normal process that promotes formation of new muscle fibers. It is often seen during early phases of training, or in growing dogs. But it is important to keep any inflammation under control so as to avoid the formation of scar tissue. To keep the inflammation down, use the cold hydrotherapy and deep massage techniques discussed later. These techniques will stir up blood circulation, bringing new oxygen and nutrients to promote healing, and break down scar tissue within the muscle fibers.

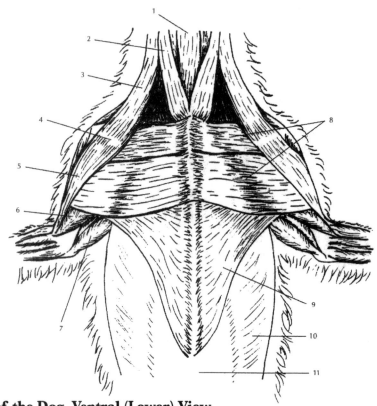

2.15 Muscles of the Dog, Ventral (Lower) View

(1) sternohyoideus muscle
(2) sternomastoideus muscle
(3) brachiocephalicus muscle, par cervicalis
(4) clavicular band
(5) cleidobrachialis muscle
(6) biceps brachii muscle

(7) triceps brachii muscle
(8) superficial pectoralis muscle
(9) deep pectoralis muscle
(10) abdominal external oblique muscle
(11) aponeurosis

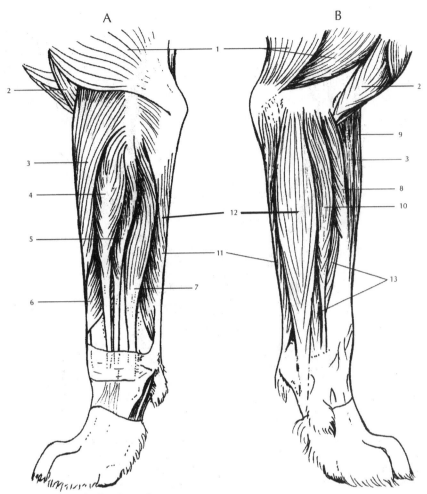

2.16 Muscles of the Foreleg

(A) Lateral
(B) Medial

(1) triceps brachii muscle
(2) biceps brachii muscle
(3) extensor carpi radialis muscle
(4) common digital extensor muscle
(5) lateral digital extensor muscle
(6) ulnaris lateralis muscle

(7) extensor carpi unlaris muscle
(8) pronator teres muscle
(9) extensor carpi radialis muscle
(10) flexor carpi radialis muscle
(11) flexor carpi ulnaris muscle
(12) superficial digital flexor muscle
(13) deep digital flexor muscle

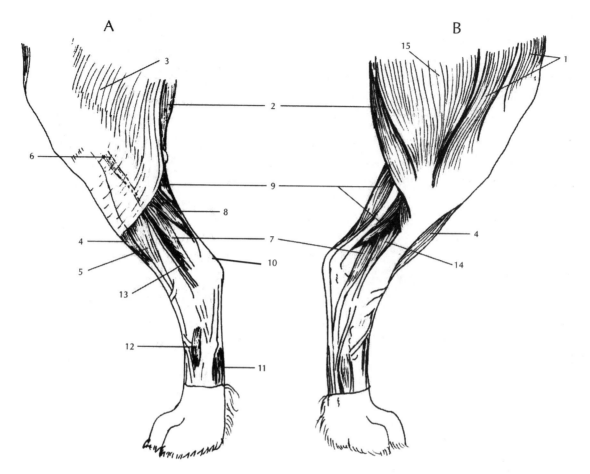

A

B

2.17 Muscles of the Hind Leg

(A) Lateral

(B) Medial

(1) sartorius muscle
(2) semitendinosus muscle
(3) biceps femoris muscle
(4) cranial tibial muscle
(5) long digital extensor muscle
(6) peroneus longus muscle
(7) deep digital flexor muscle

(8) superficial digital flexor muscle
(9) gastrocnemius muscle
(10) calcanean tendon
(11) interosseus muscle
(12) common digital extensor muscle
(13) peroneus brevis muscle
(14) lateral digital extensor muscle
(15) gracilis muscle

As a result of heavy exercise, a stress point may develop close to the origin tendon of the muscle. A stress point is a small spasm in the muscle fiber. You can keep your dog free of stress points by using the stress point treatment techniques discussed later.

Another side effect of an intense training and exercise program is the formation of trigger points. A trigger point is a combination of lactic acid build-up and motor nerve ending irritation mostly found in the fleshy part (belly) of the muscle. Trigger points can be found in any muscle of the body. Massage techniques can keep your dog free of trigger points.

Study all the muscle charts and learn about all aspects of the dog's body. Understanding the interrelation of all the components of the musculoskeletal system will contribute greatly to your expertise in understanding problems and massaging the affected areas.

The Circulatory System

The circulatory system consists of the cardiovascular system and the lymphatic system. The cardiovascular system is made of the heart, arteries and arterioles, capillaries, and veins and venules. The lymphatic system consists of a network of small vessels containing the lymphatic fluid and structures called lymph nodes which cleanse and filter.

Arterial blood circulation is generated by the pumping action of the heart (80-140 beats per minute in a normal adult dog) and the contraction of the arterial wall muscles sending blood to all body parts. The blood passes into the

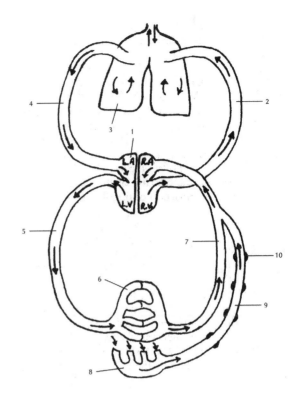

2.18 Circulatory System

(1) heart
(2) pulmonary artery
(3) lungs
(4) pulmonary vein
(5) artery
(6) capillaries
(7) vein
(8) lypmphatic capillaries
(9) lymphatics
(10) lymph nodes

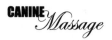

arterioles or small arteries and is distributed into the tissues via the capillaries where the oxygen/ carbon dioxide and nutrients/waste exchange occurs. The blood returns via the venule (small veins) and veins. The movement of the large locomotor muscle group of the body assists the venous return of blood. Veins are equipped with little cup-like valves to prevent the backward flow of blood. Each muscle contraction squeezes the venous blood in one direction towards the heart. The venous blood passes through the lungs where it gives up its waste as carbon dioxide gas and the red blood cells pick up oxygen from the air. Then the blood goes through the heart again and is pumped into the aorta. Blood circulation takes less than a minute to make its complete round.

Blood contains red blood cells which carry oxygen, white blood cells which fight infection and carry nutrients, and plasma, the yellowish fluid in which both of these types of cell bathe. In addition to those properties blood has several other functions, including the removal of waste products of metabolism, the transport of endocrine secretions, the equalization of water content, temperature regulation, a defense against microorganisms, immunity to disease, the blood clotting factor, allergenic reactions, and the regulation of acidity in the body.

The lymphatic system is an adjunct to the circulatory system. The lymph vessels pick up the clear, colorless fluid from the interstitial spaces (spaces between cells) that has not been returned through the venous flow. As for the venous return, the return of the lymphatic fluid is assisted by the movement of the large locomotor muscle groups of the body. Lymphatics are equipped with little cup-like valves to prevent the backward flow

of lymph. Each muscle contraction squeezes the lymphatic fluid in one direction towards the heart where it is dumped into the venous system. A series of filters - lymph nodes - prevent tissue bacteria and foreign matter from re-entering the blood stream.

The lymphatic system plays an important role in the body's defense mechanism in that it contains lymphocytes, white blood cells that aid in fighting viral and bacterial infections. Edematous swelling occurs as a result of injury, infection or other interference with the lymphatic drainage. Lack of exercise can contribute to lymphatic congestion, a condition common in older dogs.

The Respiratory System

The respiratory system includes the nose, mouth, pharynx, windpipe or trachea, bronchial tubes, bronchioles and lungs.

The lungs, somewhat elastic and filled with little sponge-like sacs known as alveoli, are where the blood gives off carbon dioxide and takes on oxygen. The diaphragm, a powerful, large and flat muscle which separates the thoracic and abdominal cavities, is responsible for the inhalation part of breathing. Exhalation is the relaxing of the diaphragm and the contraction of the rib cage muscles.

The Digestive System

The digestive system, also known as the alimentary canal, includes the mouth, the pharynx, the esophagus, the stomach, the small intestine, the colon, the rectum and anus. The digestive system alters the chemical and physical composition of food so it can be absorbed and utilized by the cells of the body. A healthy digestive tract is vital for efficient assimilation of food.

The Urinary System

The urinary system is made up of the kidneys, the ureters, the bladder, the urethra, the penis or vulva, depending on the sex of the dog.

The kidneys, by providing a blood filtering system, removes many waste products and controls water balance, pH and the level of many electrolytes. The kidney filtrate, or urine, is conveyed to the bladder by the two ureters and evacuated via the urethra.

The Endocrine System

The endocrine system is made up of glands and associated organs including the hypothalamus, pituitary, thyroid, pancreas, adrenals, liver, kidneys, spleen, ovaries or testes.

The endocrine system produces and releases hormones directly into the bloodstream. These hormones regulate growth, development and the function of specific tissues as well as coordinate the metabolic process of the dog.

The Reproductive System

The male reproductive system consists of testicles, the accessory glands and ducts, and the external genital organ. The female reproductive system consists of the ovaries, oviducts, uterus, vagina, and external genitalia. The reproductive system ensures the continuation of the species.

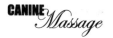

Kinesiology of the Dog

CHAPTER 3

Kinesiology is the study of motion and of the structures that make motion possible. This section is for you to use to identify the muscles involved when your animal experiences specific problems.

First, here is a list of some of the terminology that will be used.

- **Protraction:** The forward motion of the legs.

- **Retraction:** The backward motion of the legs.

- **Abduction:** The outward motion of the legs.

- **Adduction:** The inward motion of the legs.

- **Isometric contraction:** This occurs when a muscle contracts without causing an obvious movement. The best example is when a dog stands on a moving platform, like the back of a truck, and has to adjust his muscle distribution to remain standing.

- **Concentric contraction:** This occurs when a muscle shortens as it contracts and induces articular (joint) movements, such as those seen in protraction, retraction, abduction and adduction movements.

- **Agonist muscle:** When a muscle contracts it is referred to as the agonist muscle responsible for the concentric contraction.

- **Antagonist muscle:** The muscle that counteracts the agonist action is referred to as the antagonist muscle. It is elongated during the concentric contraction and is often, but not always, responsible for an eccentric contraction.

- **Eccentric contraction:** This takes place when a contracted antagonist muscle releases from its contracted state slowly to allow for better muscle control. Such a contraction permits movement to be slowed down at will. This action avoids jerky movements and allows for elegance and suppleness in the dog's movement. An eccentric contraction also acts as a shock absorber, a very important attribute during landing or any other such abrupt movement.

How a Dog Moves

To understand how a dog moves, we need to be aware of the interplay between bones, joints, ligaments, tendons and muscle groups that make the movements possible. A dog's hind legs provide the driving force and the power for the movement of the body. The forelegs are more concerned with direction and shock absorption.

Muscles are always arranged in opposing groups performing opposite actions; for example, the extensor muscle group of the foreleg extends the foot during protraction, while the flexor muscle group of the foreleg flexes the same foot during retraction. It is this type of interplay that produces the well-balanced, beautiful motion we love to see in dogs.

Protraction of the Foreleg

The muscles involved in the concentric contraction that initiates the forward motion of the foreleg are as follows:

1. The brachiocephalicus muscle.
2. The omotransversarius muscle.
3. The supraspinatus muscle.
4. The subscapularis muscle.
5. The coracobrachialis
6. The biceps brachii muscle.
7. The extensor carpi radialis muscle.
6. The common digital extensor muscle.

During protraction, the brachiocephalicus muscle pulls the shoulder joint up initiating forward movement of the foreleg. At the same time, the omotransversarius muscle pulls the ventral scapula forward while the serratus ventralis thoracis muscle contracts to assist the rotation back and downward of the top of the scapula. The supraspinatus muscle, the subscapularis muscle, the

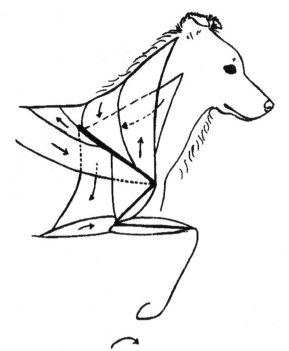

3.1 Foreleg Protraction

coracobrachialis, and the biceps brachii muscle extend the shoulder joint. The biceps brachii and mastoid muscles cause flexion of the leg at the elbow. Then the extensor carpi radialis muscle and the common digital extensor muscle extend the paw as it comes to the ground.

Also, other muscles such as the infraspinatus muscles, the thoracic part of the trapezius muscle, the deltoideus muscle and the all the pectoral muscles act as stabilizers in the protraction of the foreleg. During the protraction movement, all the muscles involved in the retraction of the foreleg are elongated and throughout their eccentric contraction ensure stability and smoothness to the movement.

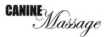

Retraction of the Foreleg

The muscles involved in the concentric contraction that initiates the backward motion of the forelegs are as follows:

1. The triceps muscle.
2. The latissimus dorsi muscle.
3. The flexor muscles.
4. The rhomboideus muscle.
5. The cervical trapezius muscle.
6. The deep pectoral muscle.

When the leg is fully protracted, the latissimus dorsi muscle and the triceps muscle are the main muscles responsible for bringing the leg backward. The deep pectoral muscle pulls backwards and towards the center of the dog, contributing to the leg retraction movement and helping prevent the leg from moving sideways. The play between the cervical and the thoracic part of the serratus ventralis muscle allows the scapula to move up and forward. The rhomboideus muscle and the cervical part of the trapezius muscle provide extra pull on the top of the scapula initiating the retraction movement. The rhomboideus also stabalizes the scapula during this movement. The flexor muscles of the foreleg provide extra push to lift the dog up and forward as the paw leaves the ground for the next stride. Also other muscles such as the supraspinatus, the infraspinatus, and the deltoideus act as stabilizers to assist the retraction of the foreleg.

All the muscles involved in the protraction of the foreleg are elongated during the retraction movement and through their eccentric contraction ensure stability and smoothness of action.

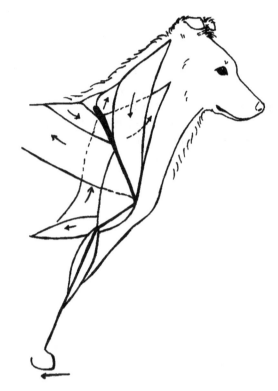

3.2 Foreleg Retraction

Abduction of the Foreleg

The muscles responsible for the concentric contraction in the abduction of the foreleg are as follows:

1. The supraspinatus and infraspinatus muscles.
2. The deltoideus muscle.
3. The rhomboideus muscle.
4. The trapezius muscle.

The elongated muscles involved in the abduction of the forelimb are as follows:
1. The deep pectoral muscle.
2. The superficial pectoral muscle.

These muscles attach along the thoracic spine and the scapula and the bones of the foreleg. Their interplay induces the abduction movement. The deltoideus, the supraspinatus and infraspinatus muscles pull the on the humerus bone laterally, bringing the leg to the outside. The trapezius and rhomboideus muscles assist this movement by pulling on the scapula up towards the top of the shoulder. The pectoral muscle group, in their eccentric contraction, contributes to the stability and smoothness of the movement.

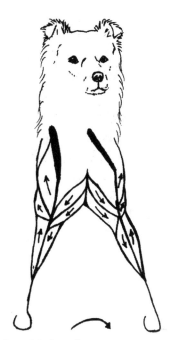

3.3 Foreleg Abduction

Adduction of the Foreleg

The muscles responsible for the concentric contraction in the adduction of the foreleg are as follows:

1. The deep pectoral muscle.
2. The superficial pectoral muscle.

The elongated muscles involved in the adduction of the foreleg are as follows:

1. The supraspinatus and infraspinatus muscles.
2. The deltoideus muscle.
3. The rhomboideus muscle.
4. The trapezius muscle.

These agonist muscles attach on the sternum and along the medial aspect of the humerus bone of the foreleg. The pectoral muscle group is principally responsible for this motion by pulling the leg medially (inward). The antagonist muscles, by their eccentric contraction, contribute to the stability and smoothness of action.

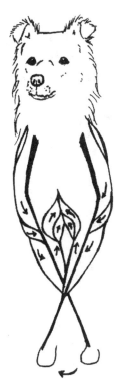

3.4 Foreleg Adduction

Protraction of the Hind Leg

The muscles involved in the concentric contraction of the forward motion of the hind leg are as follows:

1. The iliopsoas muscle (not seen in illustration).
2. The tensor fascial latae muscle.
3. The rectus femoris muscle.
4. The sartorius muscle.
5. The biceps femoris muscle.
6. The gastrocnemius muscle.
7. The extensor muscles.

The iliopsoas muscle runs deep from the inside of the pelvis to attach onto the inside aspect of the femur, below the femoral head. The ilio-

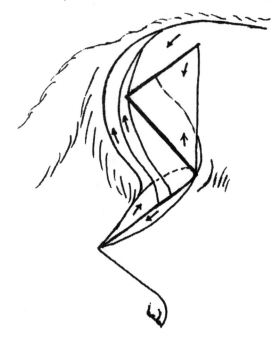

3.5 Hind Leg Protraction

psoas muscle initiates the protraction movement by pulling the femur bone up and forward. This action flexes the hip joint, the stifle joint and the hock joint. The sartorius muscle assists the iliacus by pulling the stifle up and forward. The biceps femoris muscle and the rectus femoris muscle also assist this action by pulling on the stifle joint and tibia bone, causing the stifle to flex. Also, the contraction of the gastrocnemius muscle allows the flexing of the stifle. The extensor muscles of the hind leg flex the hock joint and extend the paw.

All the muscles involved in the retraction of the hind leg are elongated during the protraction movement, while their eccentric contraction ensures stability and smoothness.

Retraction of the Hind Leg

The muscles involved in the concentric contraction of the backward motion of the hind leg are as follows:

1. The gluteus muscles, especially the middle gluteal.
2. The hamstring group (semimembranosus, semitendinosus, biceps femoris muscles).
3. The gastrocnemius muscle.
4. The deep flexor muscles.

The large middle gluteal muscle initiates the retraction movement. The hamstring muscle group is responsible for most of the power of the retraction. The gastrocnemius and the deep flexor muscles assist the flexion of the paw. The quadriceps femoris muscle assists in the extension of the hind leg at the end of the retraction movement.

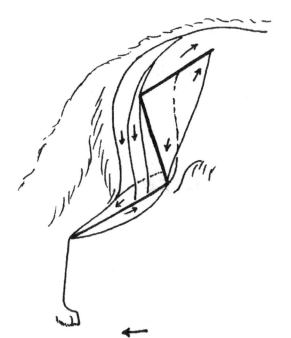

3.6 Hind Leg Retraction

The adductor muscles facilitate this motion by gently pulling the leg medially.

All the muscles involved in the protraction of the hind leg are elongated during the retraction movement, while their eccentric contraction ensures stability and smoothness of action.

Abduction of the Hind Leg

The muscles responsible for the concentric contraction in the abduction of the hind leg are as follows:
1. The middle gluteal muscle.
2. The superficial gluteal muscle.
3. The tensor fascia latae muscle.
4. The biceps femoris muscle.
5. The quadriceps femoris muscle.

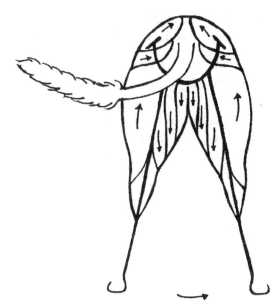

3.7 Hind Leg Abduction

The elongated muscles involved during the abduction of the hind leg are as follows:
1. The adductor muscle
   (not seen on chart).
2. The gracilis muscle.
3. The iliopsoas muscle
   (not seen on chart).

These muscles attach along the bones of the hind leg and their interplay causes the abduction movement. The tensor fascia latae muscle pulls the stifle laterally (outward). The movement is maintained by the action of the gluteus muscles, the biceps femoris, the quadriceps femoris muscle all pulling on the femur bone laterally. The antagonist muscles, by their eccentric contraction, contribute to the smoothness of action.

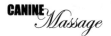

Adduction of the Hind Leg

The muscles responsible for the concentric contraction in the adduction of the hind leg are as follows:

1. The adductor muscles (not seen on chart).
2. The gracilis muscle.
3. The iliopsoas muscle (not seen on chart).

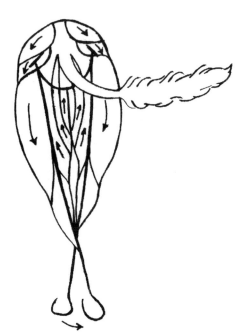

3.8 Hind Leg Adduction

The antagonist muscles involved in the adduction of the hind leg areas follows:

1. The gluteal muscles.
2. The biceps femoris muscle.
3. The quadriceps femoris muscle.
4. The tensor fascia latae muscle.

These muscles attach along the bones of the hind leg. Their interplay causes the adduction movement. The adductor muscles and the gracilis muscle are mainly responsible for this action by pulling the hind leg medially. The iliopsoas muscle assists this action. The antagonist muscles, by their eccentric contraction, contribute to the smoothness of the movement.

The Vertebral Column

In addition to protecting the spinal cord, the vertebral column provides a frame-like structure made up of strong bones and very thick ligaments. The vertibral column's role is to bridge the anterior and posterior limbs, to offer solid anchoring for the strong muscle groups and to protect the spinal cord.

Extension of the Vertebral Column

The agonist muscles responsible for the extension of the column are located above the spinal column. This extensor muscle group is made up of:

1. The spinalis dorsi muscles.
2. The longissimus dorsi muscles.
3. The iliocostalis dorsi muscles.

Flexion of the Vertebral Column

All the muscles below the spinal column are known as the column's flexors. Not only do the abdominal muscles play an important role as flexors of the spine, but so do the muscle groups involved in attaching the limbs to the spine. To some degree, the intercostal muscles assist in the flexion of the spine as well. The muscles associated with protraction, retraction, abduction and adduction of the limbs also have a second function, that of supporting the backbone.

Lateral Flexion of the Vertebral Column

Lateral flexion or bending is not caused by any specific muscle. In fact, such bending is the result of an unilateral (only one side) concentric contraction of either the flexor or extensor muscles of the spine previously mentioned. In this movement, the intervertebral muscles (not shown in illustration) play a significant role. Running from one vertebrae to the next, the intervertebral muscles are tiny muscles along each side of the vertebral column. The large oblique muscles of the abdominal group are also important in producing lateral movement.

The Rib Cage

The pectoral muscles and the serratus ventralis muscles play an essential role in supporting and stabilizing the rib cage, or chest, in relation to the spine. The abdominal muscles assist lateral bending as well as support of the rib cage. The intercostal muscles are responsible for the actual movement of the ribs. The diaphragm muscle is responsible for breathing.

The Neck Muscles

The neck muscles play a vital role in locomotion. Most obvious when running, but also seen in trotting or walking, the downward swing of the head helps to lift the rear legs off the ground as the dog moves forward. The neck muscles are as follows:

1. The splenius muscle.
2. The semispinalis capitis muscle.
3. The rhomboideus muscle.
4. The serratus ventralis cranialis muscle.
5. The trapezius muscle (cervical part).
6. The longus capitis muscle.
7. The sternohyoideus muscle.
8. The brachiocephalicus muscle.
9. The cleidobrachialis muscle.
10. The sternocephalicus muscle.
11. The omotransversarius muscle.

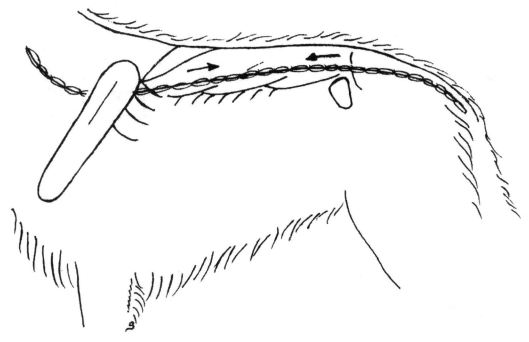

3.9 Back Extension

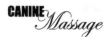

12. The intervertebral muscles
    (not seen on chart).

These muscles are attached along the spine from the base of the skull, down the cervical vertebrae to the thoracic vertebrae, to the upper ribs and the scapulas. Their interplay will induce several different movements.

Extension of the Neck

The neck muscles involved in the concentric contraction of the extension of the neck are as follows:

1. The splenius muscle.
2. The semispinalis capitis muscle.
3. The rhomboideus muscle.
4. The trapezius muscle (cervical part).
5. The serratus ventralis cranialis muscle.

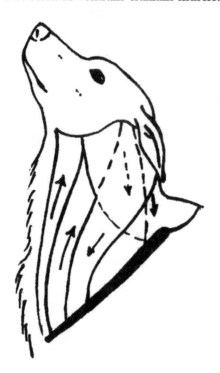

3.10 Neck Extention

As these muscles contract, they cause the cervical section of the spine to arch in extension bringing the head upwards. All the muscles involved in the flexion of the neck are elongated during the extension movement, while their eccentric contraction ensures the stability and smoothness of the movement.

Flexion of the Neck

The neck muscles involved in the concentric contraction of the flexion of the neck are as follows:

1. The sternohyoideus muscle.
2. The brachiocephalicus muscle.
3. The cleidobrachialis muscle.
4. The sternocephalicus muscle.
5. The omotransversarius muscle.

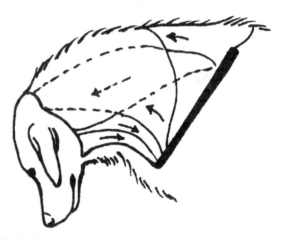

3.11 Neck Flexion

As these muscles contract, they cause the cervical section of the spine to bend forward in flexion bringing the head downwards. All the muscles involved in the extension of the neck are elongated during the flexion movement, while their eccentric contraction ensures stability and smoothness of action.

Lateral Flexion of the Neck

The lateral flexion of the neck is the result of a unilateral concentric contraction of either flexor or extensor muscles of the neck. Such unilateral contraction will cause the head and the spinal column to rotate to the same side. The play between the flexors and extensors will allow the dog to rotate upward or downward. However, the brachiocephalicus muscle and the omotransversarius

muscle are the main actors during a lateral flexion of the neck. The intervertebral muscles play a significant role in the torque of the neck. All the muscles involved on the opposite side of the neck are elongated, while their eccentric contraction ensures the stability and smoothness of the movement.

Knowing which muscles are involved in which movement will give you great confidence in your assessment and massage of the animal. This knowledge will greatly contribute to the success of your work.

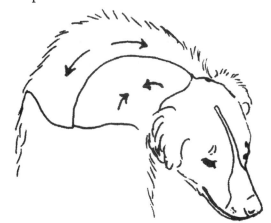

3.12 Lateral Neck Flexion

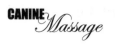

Principles and Concepts of Massage

CHAPTER 4

Massage applied with knowledge and skill not only help specific health problems in dogs, but also improves their general health and fitness. Massage has a positive influence on both the physical and psychological well-being of dogs of all ages and conditions. The caring feeling transmitted to a dog through the soothing contact of massage will contribute to the relaxation of the nervous system and assist in relieving its stress. The mechanical effect of massage on the body's tissues will increase blood circulation, improve the input of nutrients and fresh oxygen, as well as facilitate the removal of toxins. It will loosen tight muscle fibers, knots, spasms and trigger points.

Massage has a profound overall effect on animals, influencing, as it does:

• Stimulating or sedating the nervous system.

• Increasing or draining blood flow through the blood vascular system.

• Accelerating the cleansing effect of the lymph vascular system.

• Increasing oxygen/gas exchanges through the respiratory system.

• Increasing metabolic rate of the digestive system.

• Increasing fluid circulation of the urinary system.

• Increasing nutrition and flexibility of the muscular system.

• Increasing nutrition of the bone and joint structure.

After a massage therapy treatment, the "feel good" sensation derived erases much nervous tension and anxiety. This sensation will convey a sense of satisfaction and reconnection with life that subconsciously promotes recovery and improvement.

During the first massage, your dog may wonder what you are doing, but after a few sessions he will show signs of enjoyment during the massage sessions (head down, eyes almost closed, ears relaxed, etc.). When dealing with painful conditions, massage therapy has a pain relief effect on the animal. Although unproven scientifically, it is theorized that massage inhibits pain by stimulating the release of endorphins, opiate-like enzymes produced in the brain to reduce pain awareness.

The Skills of Massage

In order to develop your skills in massage, you need to understand, feel, and recognize the various elements that are part of giving a massage. The quality of your touch is most important as it delivers a soothing feeling to the dog and your touch will perceive the structures being worked on as well. In order to develop your skills in massage, consider these factors:

Proper Approach

The way you approach your dog is most important—for example being calm and aware of his personality. Review Chapter 1 for more details. A full understanding of this approach will ensure good mental and physical contact during a massage session.

Proper Posture

Your good posture is essential in giving a good massage. Good posture and proper table height help you save your energy by avoiding unnecessary movement and reducing fatigue. Review Chapter 1 for more details.

Good posture is the sum of the mechanical efficiency of the body. With good posture, you will feel well grounded in your work and more centered. You will feel your own body's energy field, as well as your dog's, and this will allow a better exchange between the two of you. With your arms and hands relaxed, you will perform the massage smoothly, avoiding tension in your chest, shoulder and back areas. As you get involved in the work, take deep breaths regularly to keep relaxed.

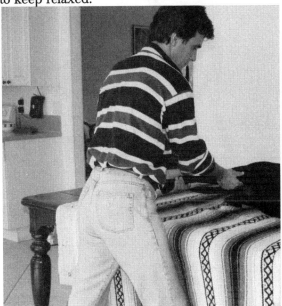

4.1 Proper Posture Standing

To maintain good posture, be sure to do the following:

• Stand with your back straight, neither rigidly nor stiffly. Your shoulders should be loose and mobile.

• Relax and breathe slowly and deeply. Adapt your breathing rhythm to that of the dog.

• Keep your head straight. Imagine a cord pulling you up lightly from the top of your head to the ground.

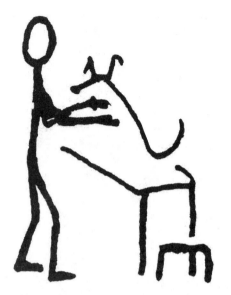

4.2 Proper Posture Standing: *Back straight elbows and knees flexed*

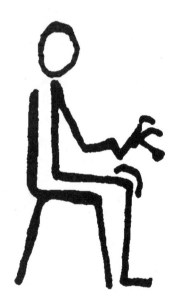

4.3 Proper Posture Sitting: *Comfortable with back straight, arm relaxed and elbow flexed*

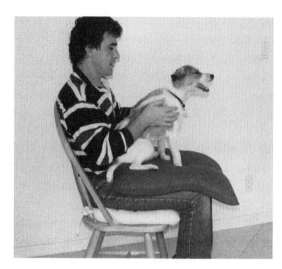

4.4 Proper Posture Sitting

- Tuck in your chin slightly.

- Look forward.

- Drop your shoulders. Do not tense the neck.

- Stretch out your arms, then let the elbows flex a little. You will now be at the right distance from the dog.

- Develop a feeling of working from your elbows, not just your hands and wrists. This action will save energy and prevent soreness. Furthermore, it will give you more strength as you will feel more connected to your whole body.

- Use your body weight when doing large movements to prevent serious fatigue.

- Bend your legs slightly at the knee, keeping your feet apart at shoulder width, similar to the Tai Chi stance.

- Be light on your feet to always be ready to move, using your full body weight in your movements. This agility will also help prevent awkward situations should the dog move unexpectedly.

- Work from your pelvis when exerting pressure; this action will help you exert more power from your body, saving tension in your arm and shoulder.

In summary, always be aware of your posture during a massage. You will maximize your energy and the quality of your treatment. With some practice, good posture will become automatic to you.

For proper posture to become second nature to you, practice mental reinforcement at the beginning of or during a treatment with a "posture check":

- Head up, chin in, look forward.

- Back straight, not stiff, breathing relaxed.

- Neck relaxed, shoulders loose, elbows flexed.

- Knees slightly flexed, feet apart at shoulder width.

- Moving and flowing from the pelvis.

With your arms and hands relaxed, good posture will allow you to perform the massage smoothly and avoid tension in your chest, shoulder and back. As you get involved in the work, take deep breaths regularly to keep relaxed. Use your body weight to regulate the amount of pressure applied. Avoid unnecessary movements of the body which will fatigue you and may annoy the animal.

Good posture will ensure an energy flow from your hands to the dog and back to you, benefiting both you and the dog. Stand fairly close to your dog to reinforce this energy exchange. It is important to give the dog the feeling of closeness to increase its relaxation and benefit from your treatment. But exercise judgment. Closeness reinforces the feeling of care that occurs naturally when giving a massage, but if the dog objects to your proximity, you should always be ready to move away.

Sensitivity of the Hands

A good touch provides a soothing and comforting feeling during your treatment. The palms of your hands and your fingertips will give you accurate feedback on the physiological state of the various parts you are working on. However, learning to trust your hands is not easy. You must concentrate so as to detect subtle changes in the body on which you are working. The quality of your work depends strongly on the sensitivity of your hands.

In the early stages of your practice, a good way to develop your perception is to work with your eyes closed. This will help you focus on your fingertips, developing your tactility ("feel-see") and enhancing your "giving" touch awareness. This manual participation in the massage has a double beneficial effect for you. First, massage stimulates the circulation of blood to your hands and fingertips, nourishing them and preventing congestion. Second, since the nerves in the fingertips are directly connected to the brain, the use

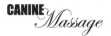

of the hands tends to promote a feeling of psychological ease. The Chinese habit of turning walnuts around and around in the hand springs from a knowledge of the salutary effect of manual activity.

The Four T's

The nerve endings in your fingers will give you considerable information about the physiological state of the body part you are massaging, helping you in your diagnosis. The sensations you perceive can be classified into four main categories: temperature, texture, tension, tenderness.

Temperature

The normal body temperature of a dog is 38°C (99 to 102°F). Changes in the temperature of the dog's skin suggest that certain problems exist. For example, an area that is abnormally cool to touch compared to the rest of the body, due to lack of blood circulation in that area, may indicate problems such as muscle contraction and/or deep chronic tension and eventually pain. An area that is hot to the touch indicates the presence of an inflammation and is a sure sign of an underlying problem such as a micro-spasm, stress points, trigger points or trauma.

Texture

Texture of the tissues refers to the density and the elasticity of the skin and muscular fibers. With practice on healthy animals, you will quickly develop a sense of touch for what normal, healthy tissues feel like. Tissues which feel either too soft or too puffy indicate the presence of swelling (edema) — a sign of congestion or of an underlying inflammatory condition.

Tenderness

Tenderness of the structures such as muscles, tendons, ligaments, joints will relate to the sensitivity response of the animal to your touch. If sensitivity is high, it is a sure sign of an underlying problem — nerve endings are irritated or perhaps damaged. The dog's reaction to your touch is proportional to the degree of severity of that condition and of its stress level.

Tension

Tension refers to the tonicity of the muscle fibers. Muscle tension is often the result of too much exercise. Sometimes, muscle tension can result from scar tissue build-up. Too much tightness means less blood circulation, less nutrients, less oxygen. Tension will increase toxin build-up, creating an underlying inflammation. Trigger points (lactic acid build-ups) and stress points (small spasms) may result. It is normal to expect some high muscle tone immediately after exercise. However, finding tension in the muscle fibers after a good rest is a sure sign of some muscular compensation problems which often develop in response to some other problem. Too much tension in a muscle may be a sign of scar tissue developing as a result of an inflammation.

Thus when you start a massage, always remember to use your fingers as sensors to get feedback through the four T's on the condition of the animal you are working on. Your fingers should become an extension of your brain. Use them as probes, quickly feeling and assessing what they touch, knowing almost instinctively how to adjust the pressure and to adapt to the right massage move. You will be amazed to find how fast this heightened perception will develop in you.

Pressure, Contact, Rhythm

The key to a successful massage is in the heightened perception of your fingers and the mastering of pressure, contact and rhythm.

Pressure

To appreciate how much pressure you are applying in a massage, experiment by pressing on a kitchen or a bathroom scale. You will be amazed to find how quickly pressure builds up. Practice by using simultaneously or alternately, one thumb, two thumbs, fingers of one hand, fingers of two hands, the palm of the hand, two palms, one fist, two fists, your elbow, etc. Then practice the various massage moves discussed later on the scale with, and without, using your body weight. Be creative! This exercise will help you realize how little exertion you need in order to reach deep into the muscle structure.

During a massage, be very careful of the pressure you exert. Too much pressure can bruise the muscle fibers without being noticed. Obviously, a bruise can't be seen under the dog's coat. The indication of a bruise will be the slight hardening of the tissues - caused by a congestion of blood - and the tenderness of the tissues that you will feel on palpation shortly after treatment.

Also, use a weight scale to practice evaluating a 1 or 3 pound pressure, then a 5 or 10 pound and up to 15 or 20 pounds. Repeat the exercise until you are aware and can feel what it takes for you to reach any desired level of pressure.

A finger stroking touch rates at 0.1 to 0.5 pound. A light touch is 0.5 to 3 pounds. A regular touch is 3 to 5 pounds. A firm touch is 8 to 15 pounds. A heavy pressure starts at 15 pounds. More than

25 pounds of pressure you can bruise fibers in muscle layers of an average animal. Use heavy pressure only on large muscle groups. If the dog has been well warmed-up, it will take the heavy pressure much more easily during the massage.

When working on scar tissue or on ligaments, use up to 25 pounds of pressure, but again be very careful at that particular stage of your massage. The best pressure is one sufficient to cause a sensation midway between pleasure and pain. A good masseur or masseuse can apply pressure that produces deep bodily effects without discomfort. When getting to the deeper aspects of your work, closely observe the animal's feedback signs, especially the eyes.

Remember, your posture should always be such that you use your body weight at all times; if necessary, you can relieve the pressure immediately. Using your body's weight will prevent fatigue of your shoulder, neck and arms.

Choosing the right degree of pressure will mostly depend on the symptoms shown by the dog (for example, if an inflammation is present or not) and by your goals in this particular massage, whether its for maintenance or to help relieve discomfort.

Always begin with a light pressure and work progressively into heavier pressure. Never jab your fingers into the animal's flesh. Start with light strokings; follow with effleurages, a gliding movement done with the palm and fingers; then build up your work with wringings, kneadings or compressions, all interspersed with effleurages every 20 to 30 seconds before using pressures above the 15 pound mark. Do not get carried away while working over stress or trigger points or on scar tissue. Very heavy pressure will trigger sore-

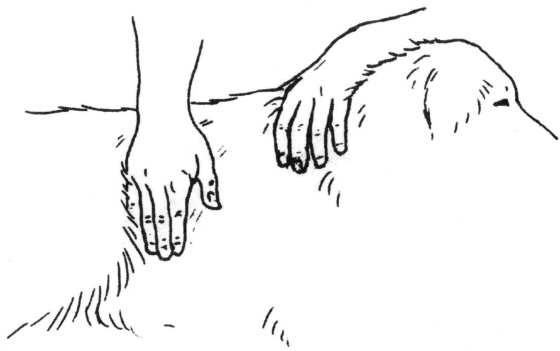

4.5 Proper Hand Contact: *Hands in full contact, molded to the part.*

ness in the muscles, especially the next day. Use the 4 T's. Always pay attention to the feedback signs of the animal, "listen" to your fingers. Pain and discomfort should always be regarded as a warning signal. Be attentive, constantly adjusting the pressure of your massage. It's better to give several light treatments than one too heavy. Consequently, always ease off progressively from heavier pressure work by using lighter wringings, general finger frictions, kneadings, and so on, all interspersed with effleurages every 20 to 30 seconds.

Contact

To get the best touch contact with the dog, keep your hands flexible, molding its body parts. Remember this is your point of contact with the animal. A mindful contact will be strongly perceived by the animal, strengthening its trust in your work. Much information passes through your hands, both to you and to the animal. You should feel a lot of warmth and lots of energy flowing through your hands during a massage. This deeper sense of contact will give you a lot of feedback on what is happening with the animal as you are progressing with your massage.

Always weave each stroke into the other to give a feeling of continuity. Never remove your hands completely before the end of a massage move. At all times, keep hand contact even when going around the dog to go on the other side. If you do not weave your moves one into another, if you often lose hand contact during the massage, you will create a disruptive feeling that prevents the dog from relaxing (you would feel the same if you were being massaged in that manner). Keeping hand contact makes a big difference in ensuring connection and comfort. Your proper posture will ensure that you work smoothly, passing on a feeling of general relaxation to the animal.

Being continually in contact during a massage, your thumbs, your fingers and your palms need careful attention. Whether employing the thumbs or the fingers, always press downward using the bulbs of the tips, not just the tips. When pressing forward with the tips you can tire or even injure your hands. Overuse of finger joints can result in premature arthritis. Because living tissues develop with use, years of correct massage action can give you well developed, silky-smooth thumbs of the kind essential to this profession.

Rhythm

In this context, rhythm refers to the frequency in which you apply your movements. Rhythm plays a strong factor in the effectiveness of your massage.

A gentle almost slow rhythm of one stroke per second is used most frequently. Use a soothing rhythm to start your session, to weave your moves into one another, and to finish your work. A soothing rhythm works wonders in relaxing the dog's nervous system, yet this soft approach allows you to work deeply if necessary. A faster rhythm stimulates the animal. It is used to perk-up the animal before exercising, to stir up circulation before deep treatment or simply to warm up your animal when it is chilled. Be aware that too brisk a rhythm could quickly irritate the dog, causing it to react against this type of massage. Always start with a gentle rhythm until you clue in on the comfortable rhythm for your dog.

The choice of specific rhythm is further discussed in the various techniques and routines outlined later. Develop your sense of rhythm by counting in your head, by listening to music or by singing.

With practice you will develop an inner appreciation of the feedback from your fingers and will know exactly how to adjust the right pressure with the right contact and at the right rhythm. Solid knowledge of the structure you are working on and of your massage techniques, plus a strong dose of common sense, is all you need to keep these three dimensions of pressure, contact and rhythm in harmony.

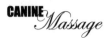

Massage Movements

CHAPTER 5

There are a number of massage movements that bring about a variety of positive effects; the most important ones will be described in this chapter.

Mechanical Effect

Mechanical effect is the actual physical contact caused by the pressure applied on the body. Therefore the mechanical effect is directly proportional to the pressure. The force you exert in the massage moves will stretch the tissues and drive the fluids (arterial, venous and lymphatic) in the direction of the movements. Light pressure will gently start things moving, whereas heavier pressure will strongly affect the area being worked on. Responding to the mechanical stimulation of the tissues, there is an increase in blood circulation in the area massaged. The results are better tissue oxygenation, better metabolism, and lowered blood pressure. Deep mechanical pressure will also contribute to the release of endorphins. Although unproven scientifically, it is theorized that massage inhibits pain by stimulating endorphin release. The mechanical pressure of specific massage moves will stretch and soften the tissues. This stretching and softening will

help release muscle tension, contractures, trigger points, stress points and spasms, eventually breaking down scar tissue.

Mechanical pressure also produces an effect on the nervous system. Depending on the type of application, it will either stimulate or soothe muscles. For example, slow, rhythmic, light-to-medium pressure will soothe and relax very efficiently, whereas faster rhythm with medium-to-heavy pressure will stimulate very quickly.

Pure Nervous Reflex Effect

The pure nervous reflex effect refers to the class of movement which influences only the nervous system. This nervous reflex effect is achieved with a very light touch. Exert almost no pressure, but rather, lightly contact the skin to touch the cutaneous sensory nerve endings. Stroking, fine vibrations and very light and slow effleurage are mostly used to elicit this nervous reflex effect. Gentle stimulation of the dermatomes - skin sensory nerve endings - sends relaxing impulses to the brain. The motor nerves, those responsible for muscular contractions or nervous anxiety, then "let go" of the tension. For this type of massage, use a slow, gentle, soothing and nourishing rhythm of one stroke per second or slower on average.

Pure nervous reflex is used primarily to soothe and relax when you need to calm your animal when it is in a state of general tension, anxiety, shock or pain (see the relaxation massage routine in Chapter 7). Pure nervous reflex does not increase the secretion of glands, cause a chemical effect, or have a mechanical impact on circulation of fluids.

Massage Moves

This section introduces the seven essential classes of massage moves and a multitude of combinations. The seven essential classes of massage moves are: stroking, effleurage, petrissage, shaking, vibration, friction and tapotements.

Each individual class contains several moves and each move can be performed in either a soothing or a stimulating manner, depending on the pressure and the rhythm applied. As a rule, the rhythm of application should be of 20 strokes per minute for a slow rhythm, and 60 strokes per minute for a gentle rhythm, 80-90 strokes per minute for a faster, stimulating rhythm. Indeed, the size of the area you massage influences the adjustment of your rhythm as when stroking a long back versus stroking short legs. Finer adjustments are specified with each class and movement.

Some of the movements appear very similar, but they all offer specifics of which you need to be aware. This knowledge will help you become an expert in choosing the right massage move to suit the necessary massage. With practice this will become second nature to you. Remember that each massage movement helps you "feel" the structures you work on and therefore gives you tremendous feedback. Due to the high sensitivity of your dog, always start lightly before increasing pressure or rhythm.

Stroking

Stroking is used for its soothing, relaxing and calming effect (pure nervous reflex effect) on the body, directly affecting the central nervous system. It is the main move used in the relaxation massage routine. When the dog is very nervous, stroking his back and legs will soothe and "ground" him.

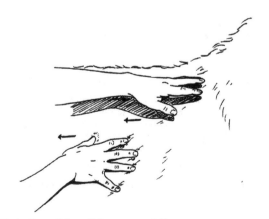

5.1 Stroking Massage Movement

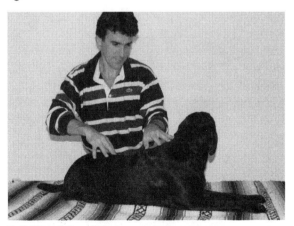

5.2 Stroking Massage Movement

You always start or finish a massage routine or treatment by applying several strokings over the body part that has been worked on. Also use strokings to weave various massage techniques or when moving from one area of the body to another.

Stroking movements are performed in a relaxed, superficial manner with the tips of the fingers or the palms of the hands, very lightly. When stroking, use very light pressure, from 0.1 to 0.5 pound pressure. This is a pure nervous reflex move, so there is no need for mechanical pressure. Stroking can be done in any direction, but preferably along the length of the muscles, following the direction in which the hair lies.

Done in slow motion, one stroke every 3 to 6 seconds on average, stroking gives a very soothing, relaxing sensation, almost sedative in its effect. Done faster, stroking will have a stimulating, almost exciting effect on the animal's nervous system.

Effleurage

Effleurage is the move you will use the most. Effleurage is used as every second move (every 10-20 seconds) during most of the massage work to emphasize proper drainage. After strokings, it is used to start, weave or terminate any massage routine or technique. To assist the natural flow of the venous blood circulation, always perform effleurage towards the heart.

Effleurage is a gliding movement done with the palmar aspect of the whole hand – the fingers and palm. During an effleurage stroke, the thumb never leads the hand but, rather, it follows the fingers. The hand should be well-molded and in full contact with the body part being massaged. You can use one or two hands, simultaneously or alternately, in an even gliding movement. The pressure is usually even throughout the entire stroke, except, for example, when going over bony processes such as the scapular ridge, point of the hip, or point of the elbow or hock.

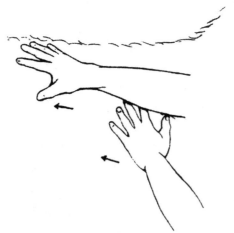

5.3 Effleurage Massage Movement

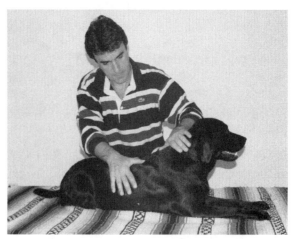

5.4 Effleurage Massage Movement

Effleurage has a mechanical, draining effect on body fluids such as blood and lymph. This draining effect is proportional to the pressure applied and the rhythm of the movement. The rhythm of your effleurages should be smooth, averaging 1 stroke every 2 or 3 seconds. A faster rhythm, 1 or 2 strokes per second is more invigorating.

When performed in a superficial manner with a light pressure and a slow rhythm, effleurage will have a very soothing effect in addition to boosting the circulation. Due to the comforting feeling it gives, this massage move is very good when starting or finishing a massage.

When effleurage is done in a similar fashion but with a faster rhythm (2 strokes per second), it is more stimulating. It can be used in this way during treatment on small areas to drain swelling without hurting the structure. But do not use this combination over a large area. The fast rhythm often causes nerve irritation and makes the dog nervous.

When effleurage is applied in a deep manner with heavy pressure and a slow rhythm, it stimulates the body by increasing blood and lymph circulation. Yet the slow rhythm still soothes the nervous system. This combination is used to drain large areas between sequences of massage moves as in the maintenance massage routine and after heavy training as discussed in more detail later.

When effleurage is done in a deep manner with faster rhythm, it strongly stimulates circulation. In this fashion, effleurage is used mostly to perk up the muscles just before exercise or as a warm up move at the end of a maintenance massage routine.

When doing effleurage on a narrow area (for example, the lower legs) use mostly the palmar region of the fingers instead of the whole hand. Adjust the pressure corresponding to the structure being worked on. Work lightly over ligaments and bony structures but more heavily over muscle groups.

Always perform effleurage toward the heart so as to assist the natural flow of the venous blood circulation.

Petrissage

Petrissage is the foundation of massage. It comprises kneading, compression, muscle squeezing, wringing-up and skin rolling.

All these moves are mechanical and soothing when done at a rhythm of 1 stroke per second, but if done at a faster rate of 2 to 4 strokes per second, they will become stimulating. The moves are intended to clean tissues of waste products and to assist circulatory interchange. Petrissage manipulations are done with pressure and relaxation alternately. With the kneading, compression and muscle squeezing massage moves, the tissues are pressed against the underlying structure. While with the wringing up and skin rolling massage moves, the tissues are lifted away from the underlying structure. Used constantly in sport massage, these moves work on muscle tension, muscle knots, congestion and small spasms.

Kneading

Kneading is a very effective technique performed with the thumbs or the palmar surface of the three fingertips (index, major and ring finger). It is done in a rhythmical, circular way—small half circles overlapping one another, pushing outwards—the same way you would knead dough. Contact is maintained at all times.

The tissues are intermittently compressed against the underlying bone structure. In a relaxing mode, the rhythm should be 1 movement per second; to stimulate, increase the rate to 2 to 4 movements per second. Kneading will have a pumping effect which boosts the circulation, improves the oxygenation and helps remove toxins from the tissues. It gives in-depth touch to the various bundles of muscle fibers, separating them, draining them and cleansing them from toxin buildup. Kneading will help you feel scar tissue patches or small spasms (stress points).

Kneading is usually performed with two hands but it may be performed with one hand when the area treated is small (the flexor tendon, for example). You can try other combinations using only two fingers or a thumb and fingers. When dealing with large areas, use the palms of your hands in combination with your body weight with proper posture. It is a very efficient technique.

When kneading, gauge your pressure. Start at 2 or 3 pounds. Increase to between 5 and 12 pounds when working the big bulky muscle groups on larger dogs. Intersperse your kneadings with a good deal of effleurages every 20 seconds.

Compression

Compression movements are made with the palm of the hand or with a lightly clenched fist, alternating each hand rhythmically and applying pressure directly onto the muscle groups. Compression is applicable to large dogs only, when working over large, bulky muscle areas such as the hind legs. The method is similar to kneadings but without the gliding movement over the muscles. The rhythm should be of one compression every

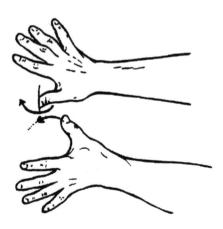

5.5 Petrissage Class of Movement: *Double Thumb Kneading*

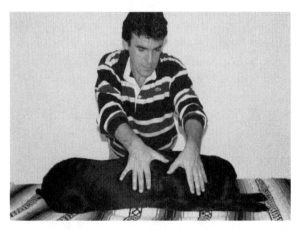

5.6 Petrissage Class of Movement: *Double Thumb Kneading*

second. Any faster would be highly stimulating, almost irritating to most animals. Do not use compression on bony or thin muscle layered areas.

Compression complements kneading; it is used to save time and reduce fatigue when working on large muscle groups. Compression produces the same pumping effect and offers the same benefits as does kneading. Be careful not to overcompress the muscles. Gauge your pressure at between 10 and 20 pounds maximum. It is better to repeat the exercise several times and secure

the desired effect than to go too fast or too heavily resulting in irritated or bruised fibers. Intersperse your compressions with a good deal of effleurages every 20 seconds.

Muscle Squeezing

Muscle squeezing is mostly used to decongest and relax tense muscles. It is used mostly along the crest of the neck and is a very useful move to work on the legs and the tail. The movement is made between extended fingers and the heal of

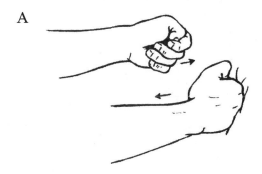
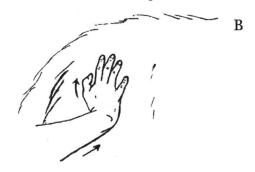

5.7 Petrissage Class of Movement:
(A) Fist Compression   *(B) Palmar Compression*

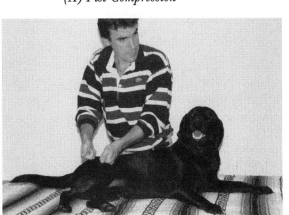
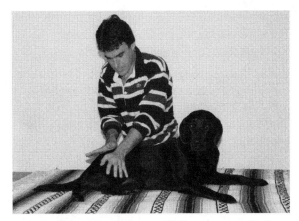

5.8 Petrissage Class of Movement: *Fist Compression*   **5.9 Petrissage Class of Movement:** *Palmar Compression*

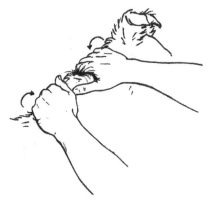

5.10 Petrissage Class of Movement:
Muscle Squeezing

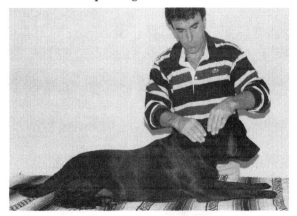

5.11 Petrissage Class of Movement:
Double Hand Muscle Squeezing

the hand using the entire palm surface in full contact with the body part. You can use one hand or two hands to deliver muscle squeezings. Taking care not to pull the muscle away from its bony support, grasp and gently squeeze it.

Muscle squeezing accomplishes several things. It gives a strong feel of touch to the animal and therefore deepens the relaxation of the muscle. It gives you feedback about the tension in these particular fibers. And it has a pumping effect on both the blood and lymph circulation.

Because the goal with this move is to relax and decongest, it is not necessary to exert a lot of pressure in this move. When muscle squeezing, always start gently with 5 to 10 pounds pressure. You can use 15 pounds pressure if dealing with bulkier muscle groups of larger dogs such as thicker neck, legs or pectoral muscles. But remember, if there is tenderness in the muscle, squeeze very gently.

Using muscle squeezing in a soothing, slow rhythm (1 squeeze every second) has a strong calming effect on the nervous system. It is used for this purpose in the relaxing massage routine, over the neck. When done in a brisk manner, double hands muscle squeezing has a very stimulating effect both on the circulation and on the nervous system. The fast pace invigorates the animal. It is a very useful move to warm up the leg muscles such as the triceps, the flexors and extensors of the legs during cold weather.

Wringing Up

Wringing up is a great move to use on the back of the dog, the shoulders and hind quarters. Wringing up efficiently increases the circulation,

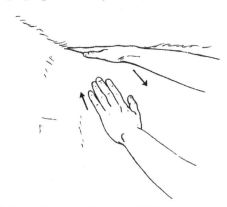

5.12 Petrissage Class of Movement:
Wringing

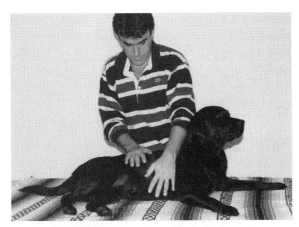

5.13 Petrissage Class of Movement:
Wringing

improves the oxygenation and removes toxins. It is very useful in reducing inflammation over the muscles of the back and dogs love it!

Wringing up is done with the palmar surface of the hand, thumbs abducted at a 90° angle. Apply both hands flat on the body part then start wringing the muscle side to side, almost in the same way you would wring wet linens. The muscle is lightly and gently lifted then wrung side-to-side.

Wringing up is very efficient in stimulating the circulation and warming up muscle groups in a short time. Wringing up can be applied anywhere on the dog's body. Use an average pressure, starting at about 2 pounds and building up to 15 pounds depending on the muscle mass worked on. Remain light when going over bony areas such as the spine, the scapula or point of the hip. Your rhythm should be smooth, 1 stroke per second or less on average. A faster rhythm of 2 strokes per second will be very stimulating and may be irritating to the dog.

Skin Rolling

Skin rolling is a very soothing manipulation which is used mostly to keep the dermal layer rich in blood. Skin rolling is used mostly to maintain a healthy and shiny coat, break down little fatty deposits, prevent the formation of excess adhesions and maintain good elasticity of the skin.

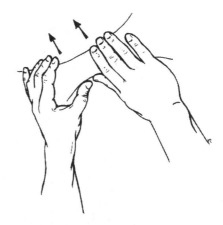

5.14 Petrissage Class of Movement:
Skin Rolling

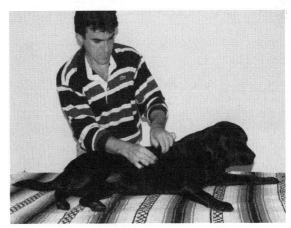

5.15 Petrissage Class of Movement:
Skin Rolling

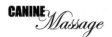

With thumbs on one side and fingers on the other, grasp and lift the tissues. Using either one or both hands (preferably both), push the thumbs forward rolling the skin toward the fingers. The fingers draw the skin towards the thumbs, lifting, stretching and squeezing the tissues.

Skin rolling is a gliding motion of the superficial tissues which include skin and fat. It should be performed in a slow, soothing manner to avoid irritating the skin nerve endings, especially over areas where the tissues lie tight on the underlying structures. The angle of direction may be varied and repeated to ensure maximum effect to the tissues. This is a great technique to enhance nerve and blood circulation. Skin rolling motion is used in acupuncture to stimulate the bladder meridian. When applying skin rolling, use only 2 or 3 pounds pressure maximum!

Vibrations

This interesting manipulation is mostly used to reach below superficial tissues into the deeper structures of muscles or joints. It is a quivering type of movement done with the hand. It has a soothing effect and can be used alone or inserted into a routine or treatment.

At the start, use no pressure other than the weight of your hand on the part to be vibrated, a half pound maximum. Progressively increase your pressure by a few pounds to the point of stretching the structure you are treating. Start the vibration movements from the elbow and translate them through your wrist to your hand, this is known as a "flat hand vibration."

You can use another variation called the "point vibration". This is done with the thumb or the fingertips only, giving you more accuracy for small specific areas. The aim is to pass a soothing vibration to the tissues deep under the skin.

Done gently with 1 or 2 pounds of pressure and applied with a fine, gentle rhythm, vibrations have a mechanical soothing effect with a strong nervous reflex effect. Applied with 3 to 5 pounds of pressure and a faster, more aggressive vibrational rhythm, vibrations are a mechanically stimulating move and less of a nervous reflex.

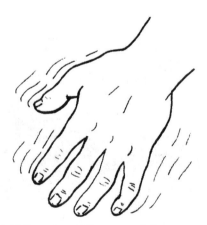

5.16 Vibration Massage Movement

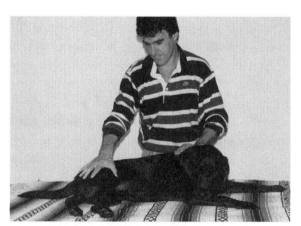

5.17 Vibration Massage Movement

This manipulation is very useful in relaxing the nervous system. Use the flat hand vibration move in a gentle manner with light pressure over the sacrum for a few minutes when starting the relaxation routine. It is very efficient in eliciting the parasympathetic nervous response. But it is not recommended to use this move directly over the skull. Apply vibration to joint spaces and around bony prominences. It soothes swollen joints both in the cases of acute trauma and chronic injury. Vibrations are also good for inflamed arthritis where regular massage is contra-indicated. Use vibrations near well-healed scar tissue so as to reduce adhesions. Depending on the area, apply no more than 5 to 10 pounds pressure until the animal's maximum tolerance is reached.

Start with a small vibratory movement, maintaining it for a few seconds. Then gradually release and move to another position. Start again and repeat over the whole area you want to treat. Intersperse effleurage and stroking frequently with this move so as to drain the tissues and relax the animal.

Shaking

Shaking is a very strong mechanical movement used frequently in sport massage to stimulate circulation. Shaking is performed either by the fingertips or with the whole palm of the hand in full contact with the body part. The skin is shaken over the muscle structure. It can either be a short shaking, over a small area, or a large shaking, over a larger area.

When done in a gentle manner at 1 stroke per second, shaking is soothing. When applied more briskly at 2 or 3 strokes per second, it is one of the most stimulating massage moves.

Pressure should be kept between 3 and 5 pounds. The skin can move with your hands over the body parts. When working more coarsely (heavier pressure, faster rhythm), the hands glide over the skin. As you work in this manner, pay attention to your animal's feedback signs. Take care not to irritate the nerve endings of the skin, especially if an inflammation is present. Adjust your rhythm and pressure accordingly. Always ease off a little when going over bony processes such as the point

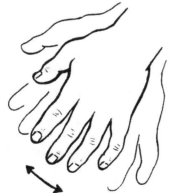

5.18 Shaking Massage Movement

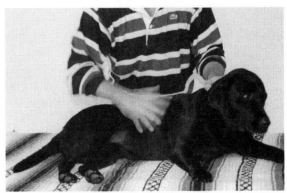

5.19 Shaking Massage Movement

of the hip or the scapular spine. A full treatment of this move alone should not exceed three to five minutes depending on the size of the dog.

Friction

This very specific movement is mostly used in sport therapy to break down adhesions developing over muscular fibers, tendons, ligaments, fas-

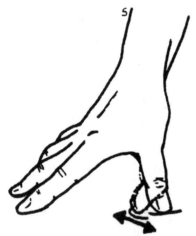

5.20 Thumb Friction Movement

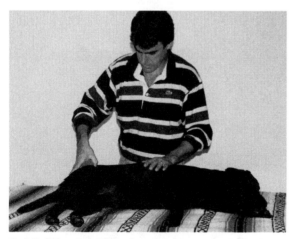

5.21 Thumb Friction Movement

cia, joint capsules and bones. Always warm up the area thoroughly with effleurages, wringing up and kneadings before proceeding to frictions.

Frictions consist of small, deep movements applied across the length of the muscle fiber bundle or up and down over a patch of fibrous tissue. Use the tip of your thumb or first three fingers to friction small, local areas. Use both hands to friction large areas. With any of these friction movements, expect to see a lot of loose fur being removed.

Friction can be done gently or coarsely depending on your aim. Both styles are mechanically stimulating to the body, causing a very strong hyperaemia response (increased blood circulation). Keep in mind the degree of tissue inflammation present, the dimension of the adhesions and their location in relation to other structures - is it close to a bone, joint, nerve or vein?

To break down fibrous adhesions, you need to use a fair amount of pressure, starting around 10 to 15 pounds, progressively building up to a maximum of 25 pounds. Always warm up the area thoroughly before starting. Your rhythm can be of 1 or 2 strokes per second for slow frictions, up to 4 frictions per second for fast frictions. When using the heavier pressure, always keep the friction movements smooth and fast. Do not use friction on one specific area for too long. At any given time, 2 to 3 minutes is enough up to a maximum of 4 or 5 minutes if no inflammation is present. It is better to reduce scar formation over the course of several massages than to take the risk of worsening the area by overworking it and creating more inflammation. It is very important to intersperse your work with copious drainage every 20 seconds and some wringing up to keep the tissues warm.

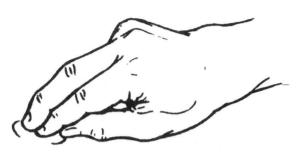

5.22 Finger Friction Movement

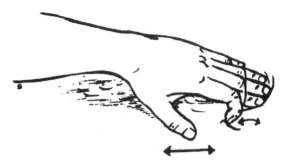

5.24 Finger Friction Movement

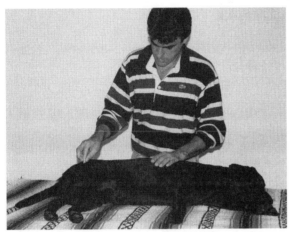

5.23 Finger Friction Movement

When working a patch of scar tissue, start from the periphery towards the center of the scar with fairly low pressure to loosen the fibers. Drain thoroughly with effleurages then use friction across the whole fibrous patch, going sideways or up and down depending on the nature of the scar formation. Follow this with a circular motion using a much heavier pressure. Assess the feedback signs of the dog. Remember to drain generously with effleurages every 20 seconds.

As you use friction to relieve new adhesions or to breakdown old ones, it is good to ice before and after treatment. This will ensure the numbing of the nerve endings and will therefore keep

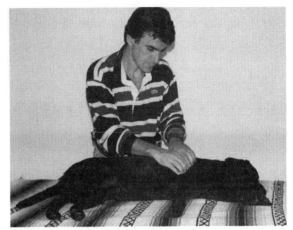

5.25 Finger Friction Movement

the pain down. Simply apply a cold pack or use the ice massage technique as described in Chapter 10.

Tapotements

Tapotement massage consists of a series of soft blows to the body done rhythmically. Tapotements comprise clapping, cupping, hacking, and beating. All these movements are mechanical and stimulating. Hands usually work alternately in a light and springy manner.

The rhythm of application varies according to the pressure. Light clapping, cupping and hacking are done at approximately 2 to 3 beats per sec-

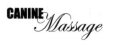
ond for starters, up to 5 beats per second when warm. The heavier beating and pounding movements are performed more slowly at 2 to 3 beats per second. The moves are mostly used to stir up circulation, to stimulate the release of histamine and to energize the body; they are used frequently in therapeutic massage treatments, sport massage sessions and in warm up routines.

Done on their own, tapotements are very effective for warming up muscle groups just prior to exercise. Your dog may take some time to adapt to

tapotements, but he will soon learn to like them. Start with a very light pressure, increasing progressively. The application of tapotements should last a few minutes: 30 seconds to one minute over small areas, up to 2 minutes when working large parts. A strong, soothing feeling of relaxation will follow such an application. Try it on yourself and you will see. Always finish with some effleurages and strokings.

Clapping

Clapping is done with the palm of the hand, the hand flat and the fingers stretched as though applauding.

Use only 2 or 3 pounds to start, building up to 5 or 10 pounds pressure. Use only on muscle groups, not on bony structures, except over the rib cage. Keep the pressure light over thin muscles like the scapular muscles.

Cupping

Cupping is done with the palm of the hand cupped as though holding water.

Use 5 pounds pressure. This is a softer version of clapping, mostly for adapting your hands around bony structures like the scapula and hip areas, or curved muscle areas like the front chest or rump.

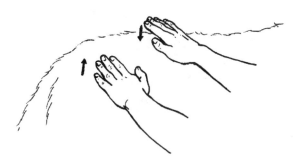

5.26 Tapotement: *Clapping Movement*

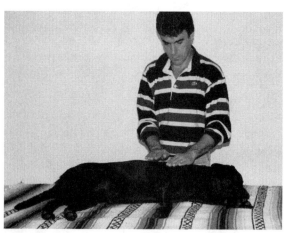

5.27 Tapotement: *Clapping Movement*

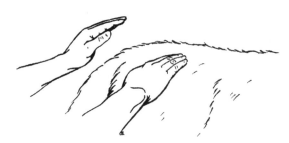

5.28 Tapotement: *Cupping Movement*

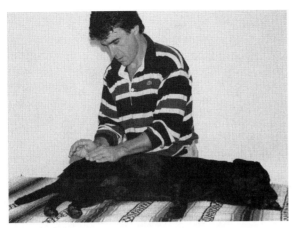

5.29 Tapotement: *Cupping Movement*

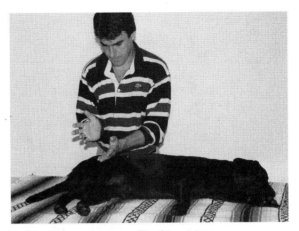

5.31 Tapotement: *Hacking Movement*

Hacking

Hacking is done in a springing manner with the medial border of the hand and the fingers spread out in a flexible and non-rigid manner.

Use 5 to 8 pounds of pressure and up to 12 pounds when working over big bulky muscles. Hacking penetrates deeper into the muscle structure and yet is very gentle. It is a favorite move to treat the back muscles (longissimus dorsi & iliocostalis dorsi) or the thicker muscle of the hind quarters.

Beating

Beating is done with a relaxed clenched fist, hitting the muscle groups with the ulnar (or medial) side of the hand.

Pressure can be of 10 to 15 pounds and up to 20 pounds over big muscle groups. Only use this move after you have already done several clapping, cupping and hacking moves. This move is rarely used except for deep stimulation of

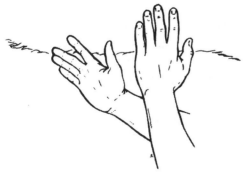

5.30 Tapotement: *Hacking Movement*

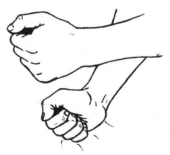

5.32 Tapotement: *Beating (medium pressure) and Pounding (heavy pressure) Movements*

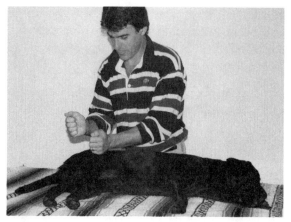

5.33 Tapotement: *Beating and Pounding Movements*

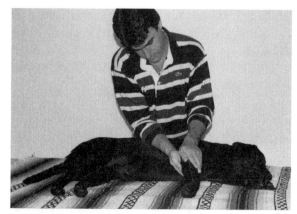

5.35 Laying On of Hands

big muscle groups like the hind quarters on big dogs. A strong stimulation of fluid circulation will immediately follow this application.

The Laying On of Hands

The laying on of hands has great therapeutic value in soothing acute wounds, inflammation, nerve irritation, stress of mechanical or nervous origin and emotional frustration. The laying

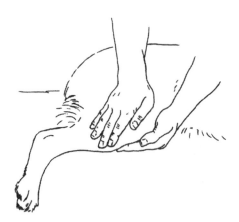

5.34 Laying On of Hands

of hands is not considered a technical massage movement in most classical massage manuals, but it is the oldest form of massage and its benefits make it a must for all therapists. The technique is mostly used where regular massage cannot be used; it is a great addition to regular treatment routines and furthers the soothing effect.

Put your hands gently over the area of concern and mindfully feel the energy and the vibration of that part. Use very little pressure—less than 1 pound—for this simple hand contact. Be thoughtful of the moment, of the animal and of yourself as you do this. The feeling of closeness that will quickly develop between you and the animal is a sure sign of the effectiveness of this procedure. A warm feeling will develop between your hands. As the nervous stress connected to that particular area is released, you will feel a heat wave coming out of the treated area. That heat wave will be proportional to the stress recorded and the pain involved. The laying on of hands will soothe the area and induce relaxation both on the physiological and the nervous levels. A great feeling of relief will follow such a procedure.

When massage is contra-indicated, the laying on of hands will often bring soothing energy to an irritated area, relieving pain. It is recommended that you rinse your hands with fresh water after such treatment, to drain the "off" energy you picked up. Cold hydrotherapy (such as a simple cotton towel wrung out of cold water) applied onto the animal's treated body part will also relieve the inflammation and pain considerably. The laying on of hands will definitely comfort your animal and assist its recovery.

Basic Classifcation of Massage Movements

Massage is classified into three basic groups: soothing, stimulating and pure nervous reflex.

Soothing Massage Movements

The main characteristic of a soothing massage is its ability to inhibit nerve impulses to the muscles soothing them into relaxation.

The soothing massage moves are as follows:

- Slow stroking.
- Gentle wringing.
- Gentle effleurage.
- Fine vibration.
- Fine shaking.
- Gentle petrissage with kneading, muscle squeezing, wringing up and eventually gentle compressions - all done with very light pressure and a peaceful rhythm.

Stimulating Massage Movements

The main characteristic of a stimulating massage is that it causes a nerve exciting reflex in the muscles. This reflex stimulates muscle tone (light con-

traction) causing an increase in blood and lymph circulation with resultant increased oxygenation, improved nutrient intake and better removal of toxins and metabolic waste.

Rhythm and pressure play important roles in the degree of stimulation you want to induce. Working in a hasty manner with a fast rhythm and abrupt changes of movement will irritate your animal very quickly. Therefore, always start gently and build up your pressure and rhythm accordingly. Always pay attention to the feedback signs of the animal. Pressure need not be heavy. On a healthy structure, 10 to 20 pounds is plenty. The mechanical repetition of the movements will secure the effects desired. Always start lightly and monitor the feedback signs of your animal, adjusting accordingly.

In time and with practice you will develop a sense for the amount of pressure and the appropriate rhythm. You should always stay on the safe side by starting gently. As your dog becomes accustomed to the massage, it will allow you to work deeper especially if it is well warmed up. Always remember to ensure thorough drainage through effleurage after using stimulating moves.

The stimulating moves are as follows:

- Fast stroking.
- Firm to vigorous effleurage.
- Petrissage with firm kneadings, compressions, wringing up and skin-rolling.
- Coarse vibrations.
- Coarse shaking.
- Frictions, fine and coarse.

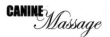

- Nerve manipulation with nerve pressure, nerve friction and nerve stretching.
- Tapotements with clapping, cupping, hacking, and beating.

Pure Nervous Reflex Movements

The main characteristics of pure nervous reflex massage moves are that they induce reflex effects on the central nervous system and result in a "let go" of nervous tension, stress and anxiety. Pure nervous reflex promotes strong relaxation.

The pure nervous reflex moves are as follows:

- Stroking.
- Very gentle effleurage.
- Fine vibrations.
- Laying of hands.

It is strongly recommended that you wash your hands with fresh water immediately after any massage work. Washing helps you unload all undesired residual energy picked up during the massage and avoids passing it on to other persons or animals. It will also center your vital energy before further activity.

Regular practice of massage on your dog, or dogs, will quickly develop your ability to feel the right approach for each type of massage. The enhanced perception of your fingertips will surprise you tremendously. You will be amazed at how much information you pick up and this, in turn, will help you appreciate the situation at hand. Remember, practice makes perfect. And even more, quality practice makes perfect!

Massage Techniques

CHAPTER

6

Massage techniques refer to specific massage moves arranged in a pattern and done in an orderly fashion to achieve a desired effect. These techniques can be applied to any body part and at any given time after proper warm up of the structures to be worked on, unless massage is contra-indicated.

The massage techniques in this chapter have been developed to further your knowledge and to provide you with guidelines for the best course of treatment in dealing with muscular problems. These techniques will prevent aggravation of those problems, speed up the healing process and ensure proper recovery.

Massage therapy has developed several deep massage techniques to eliminate muscle tightening and prevent toxin build-ups. Muscle tightening causes muscle resistance to the natural motion of the body parts resulting in, for example, a shorter stride or restricted neck movement. It will lead to the build-up of stress points, trigger points (lactic acid build-up), and congestion of fluid circulation which in turn will cause pain and potential lameness in the dog.

These techniques are as follows:

- The SEW/WES technique to start and finish any massage work.

- The thumb technique for a variety of effects.

- The swelling technique to deal with edema.

- The trigger point technique to deal with lactic acid build-up.

- The stress point technique to deal with small spasms.

- The origin/insertion technique to deal with chronic muscle contracture and full muscle spasms.

These techniques can be used separately or in any combination to ensure efficient overall treatment and positive results. Though we often use the swelling and origin/insertion techniques in emergencies, all are used in maintenance and preventive routines according to the dog's level of play or training.

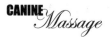

Here, more than anywhere else, the four T's apply—temperature, tension, texture, and tenderness. Every stroke will give you feedback on the condition under your fingertips. So "listen" to your fingers and adjust accordingly.

The SEW/WES Technique

This technique is very important in massage work. It gives you the proper approach for warming-up and for draining any area you wish to work on. The title of this technique is made up of two acronyms. The acronym SEW stands for Stroking, Effleurage and Wringing, while the acronym WES stands for Wringing, Effleurage and Stroking.

The SEW approach is used to start and progressively warm up any area you are to massage. Always start with very light and gentle strokings over the area you will be massaging. Then follow with two to three effleurage passes to thoroughly cover the entire area all along draining towards the heart. Now apply gentle wringings - two passes back and forth - over the whole area. Follow with a set of effleurages and continue with either kneadings, muscle squeezing and/or gentle friction depending on the nature of the massage you want to give. Remember to intersperse with effleurages every 20 seconds.

The WES approach is used when you are finished with the deeper aspect of the massage. This approach will allow you to properly and progressively move out of the area you worked on, ensuring proper drainage. After the last set of effleurages, following your deeper massage work, apply a gentle but firm set of wringings over the entire area worked on (2 passes back and forth). Follow with extra effleurages (twice as many as usual, 4 to 6 passes) to thoroughly drain

the tissues you have massaged. With each effleurage pass you should release your pressure a little, starting around 6 pounds and ending with 3 pounds. Then finish with a light stroking, covering the entire area.

The last bit of stroking in the WES approach can become the opening stroke of the SEW approach to the area you will massage next.

The Thumb Technique

The thumb technique plays a very important role in massage movements, in palpations and in assessing the structures to be treated. Due to its shape, strength and versatility, the thumb is a key player in most of your massage moves. It is your most valuable tool for deep work (friction of adhesions).

When using the thumb, form a 90° angle between it and the spread fingers. You can use the tip of the thumb like a probe or you can use the tip's medial or lateral aspects to make contact with angled surfaces.

The thumb technique is very useful when performing specific and localized work. Never use the thumb without warming up the area treated with strokings, effleurages, kneadings, and so on. For more general, less localized, less specific work, you can use the broader surface of the thumb's last phalange. The thumb's extreme malleability allows you to modify the direction of your movement as well as the force you are using at any moment depending on the signs and symptoms of the area being treated. Thus a wide range of therapeutic effects are possible. You can use the thumb to drain small or localized areas, stretch fibers, friction scar tissue,

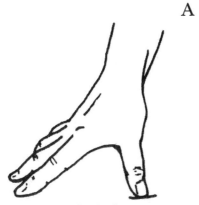 A

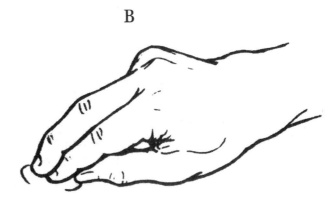 B

6.1 Thumb Technique

(A) Thumb Technique
(B) Reinforced Index Finger Technique

release trigger points and make investigative palpations and assessments. The thumb is not to be used mechanically across the tissues but is to be applied intelligently with knowledge of the structures being treated.

Because of its highly developed nervous sensory endings, your thumb sends messages directly to your brain. If you close your eyes during your thumb palpations or, during any other work, you will feel minute changes in the tissues.

To maximize your strength when using the thumb during frictions or when applying deep pressure, use your body weight. You should feel the force going in a straight line from the shoulder, through the elbow, the thumb and to the target. Allow the elbow or the wrist to bend only a few degrees. Proper posture will facilitate your work and save your energy. The level of pressure used with the thumb depends on the pathological condition of the tissues treated, the nature of the work and the location of the treatment. Use your judgment, but remember that over 25 pounds of pressure may cause bruising in muscular tissues.

If your thumb is not strong enough, you can resort to using your index finger, reinforced with your thumb and middle finger (see Figure 6.1) following the same procedure as the thumb technique.

The Swelling Technique

This technique is used to reduce swelling resulting from either acute or chronic injuries. A trauma such as a strain, sprain, wound, kick, inflammation from overwork or the flare up of an old injury will cause an increased amount of fluid (lymph or blood) to the area, resulting in swelling. This increased volume of fluid will cause an increased tension of the tissues and skin rendering them very tender to the touch. The temperature of the swollen area will be higher than normal and proportional to the degree of inflammation. Remember that any acute phase of trauma is contra-indicated to massage and that you should contact your veterinarian to ensure no other tissue damage is involved. When massage is contra-

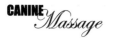

indicated, use cold hydrotherapy instead until the initial swelling goes down, then apply this massage technique.

The swelling technique should be preceded by the application of hydrotherapy as described in Chapter 10 - cold in acute cases, vascular flush (hot/cold) in sub-acute cases and heat in chronic cases. Choose the most practical device (ice packs, ice cup) available to you and apply it before your massage treatment to induce a vaso-constriction of the tissues and numbing effect of the nerve endings. The ice cup massage is a terrific, practical technique to use with swellings.

Start with some light stroking moves over the body to relax the animal and help it accept your working close to the problem site, then apply your light strokings over the swollen area to soothe the irritated nerve endings. Your rhythm

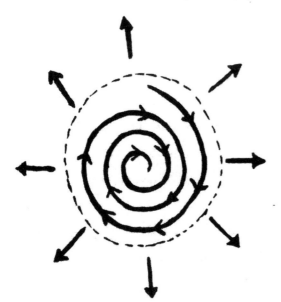

6.2 Schematic Diagram of Swelling Technique

should be smooth, 1 stroke per second. Assess the feedback signs of your dog at all times. If the area appears very irritated, use the laying on of hands approach or cold hydrotherapy before proceeding.

When the initial tenderness seems to be relieved, you can use a fine vibration movement to stimulate the circulation, then resume the light strokings. Weave your stroke into a very light effleurage—a maximum of 2 or 3 pounds pressure to avoid mechanical stress on the skin and deeper tissues—around the periphery of the swollen area, draining toward the heart. This will stimulate the circulation and begin the drainage process. Keep a relaxed pace of 1 move per second.

Next proceed with a very gentle double-thumb kneading massage at the edge of the swelling, going around the damaged area in a clock-wise manner. Drain the excess fluid towards the outside of the swollen area, "shaving" half to 1 inch from the periphery. Always start on the outside, not at the center. Use 3 to 5 pounds pressure or less if the skin is very tight or tender. Even when light pressure is used, the mechanical effect will be sufficient to rapidly induce drainage. Keep assessing your dog's feedback and speak soothing words as you proceed.

After you have completed the first circumference around the swollen area, use several light effleurages, draining away from the periphery of the trauma and always moving toward the heart.

Repeat the kneading technique, progressing in a spiral fashion towards the center of the problem area, shaving half to 1 inch at a time. Alternate with effleurages at the completion of each kneading circle around the swollen area.

During the first application of the swelling technique to a traumatized area in the acute phase (first 24 hours), leave the dead center - 1 inch diameter or more if needed - of the swelling site alone, because it is important to let the natural healing process take its course.

After the first 24 hours, the clotting of the bruised fibers will have taken place and you will be safe to massage the entire area with this swelling technique.

When in the chronic stage, after 72 hours, it is recommended that you apply some gentle frictions over the entire area to loosen and breakdown adhesions to maintain maximum flexibility between the muscle fibers, fascia and skin. Always monitor the feedback of your dog especially when doing such work. When there is considerable decrease in the swelling, use more effleurage progressively adding a little more pressure but never in a heavy manner. You may slightly increase the rhythm of your moves. Estimate the degree of inflammation and tenderness and adjust your pressure and pace accordingly.

At the end of your massage treatment, apply cold hydrotherapy again to reduce nerve irritation and encourage vasoconstriction to further assist the drainage process. The cold application's secondary effect will contribute to even out the overall circulation of fluids in that particular area.

Duration of Application

The time frames given here apply only for the massage part of the swelling technique, not the hydrotherapy application. Over a small area of 2 or 3 inches in diameter, the massage should not last more than 5 minutes in order to avoid irrita-

tion of the dermatomes. Over a larger area, 10 to 15 inches in diameter, the application should last no more than 10 minutes. If the swollen area is very large, several feet in diameter, for example a whole leg or hind quarter, do not exceed 15 minutes. Use palmar kneading instead of thumb kneading to cover more surface area. Remember that the tissues are very tender and a gentle pressure is enough to mechanically reroute the excess fluid. Always keep a relaxed rhythm of 1 move per second.

Lower Leg Swelling

When dealing with the swelling of the lower leg, first gently but thoroughly massage the upper leg so as to stir up the circulation and clear the way before pushing the excess fluid upward. Ice massage does wonders for lower leg edema. When dealing with the foreleg you can flex the elbow to bring the lower leg horizontal with one hand and work the tendon thoroughly with the other hand using mostly effleurage moves. Here your overall treatment should not exceed 20 to 25 minutes.

Follow this swelling technique with a cold hydrotherapy application, discussed later, to reduce the nerve irritation and to encourage vasoconstriction to further the drainage process. The secondary lasting vasodilatation effect of the cold application will regulate the overall fluid circulation.

Frequency of Applications

The degree of inflammation present in the tissues will determine the frequency of your treatments. Evaluate the condition by checking the degree of swelling, the temperature level of the inflammation and the level of tenderness present. It is best to do several small treatments in the course of a few days to achieve a steady rate of recovery. By attempting large, extensive treatments in a short period you risk aggravating the inflammation and delaying the healing process.

If the inflammation is very strong in a small area, apply the swelling technique only once or twice a day 10-12 hours apart; if on a large area, just once a day. You can, however, apply cold hydrotherapy several times a day for ten minutes at a time. If the inflammation is moderate, the swelling technique can be repeated two or three times a day with a minimum of 6 hours between treatments. When dealing with a larger area such as a leg, you may work this technique twice daily. As the swelling goes down and the tissues become less tender, you can use a little more pressure and more effleurages. Be gentle and very careful in the acute stage, becoming more invasive gradually as the swelling heals. Remember to use hydrotherapy before, after, and in between the treatments to accentuate the drainage process and reduce the inflammation of the nerve endings.

In the case of the flare-up of an old injury, the relief of the swelling may take twice as many treatments as in an acute injury, due to the chronic, recurrent aspect of the inflammation. If tenderness is present in the tissue, the use of cold hydrotherapy may be more beneficial than heat. But if the nerves do not appear to be irritated, use heat or vascular flush (see Chapter 10). Once the swelling is definitely gone, resume a regular massage practice.

Trigger Point Technique

The trigger point technique is used to release and drain trigger points. A trigger point forms primarily as the result of toxin build-up (mostly lactic acid). Because of the toxicity in the fibers, an irritation of the local motor nerve endings develops. The term "trigger point" originates from the fact that pressure applied to that particular point will send a pain referral to other body parts. This referred pain is mostly caused by the presence and association of nerve endings throughout the muscle groups.

A trigger point is usually found in the belly part of a muscle. Depending on your dog's level and type of activity, trigger points can form in several muscles anywhere in the body. This condition occurs mostly in response to muscle tension due to overuse or nervous stress; it is sometimes due to a lack of activity resulting in sluggish circulation. The hypertonicity or hypotonicity of the muscle fibers causes a decrease in

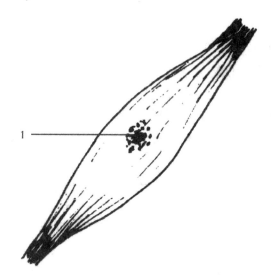

6.3 Schematic Diagram of a Trigger Point

(1) Toxin buildup in the belly of the muscle, resulting in a trigger point

blood circulation as well as a decrease in oxygen, resulting in a build-up of toxins. The increase in toxin in one particular area will trigger a nerve ending irritation.

Muscular tension is mostly due to overwork or overplay and not enough stretching or rest. Excess fatigue, nervous stress, restlessness or boredom can trigger the same muscular tension.

When the referred pain is of weak intensity, it is termed a "silent trigger point." One which sends strong sensations and is very sensitive to the touch is referred to as an "active trigger point." Frequently, trigger points are found within symptom referral areas. Occasionally, one trigger point will have more than one referral area; these are called spill-over areas.

Trigger points feel like small nodules but they occasionally can appear as larger nodules; in any size, they are usually very tender. Trigger points give easily under pressure and release fairly quickly. Hot hydrotherapy application over the specific area will contribute greatly to the effectiveness of your trigger point technique. It will loosen the tissue fibers and boost the circulation in the area. Use hot packs or hot towels. Start with the SEW approach to warm up the muscles. Then use thumb kneadings to loosen the muscle fibers and locate the area of most congestion and tenderness.

When you find the trigger point, be gentle. Use a light pressure as you apply your thumb directly over the nodule. Hold the pressure until the muscle relaxes. The release process may take just a few seconds for recently formed trigger points, or 1 to 2 minutes for more chronic trigger points. Follow the release with lots of effleurages to insure proper drainage of this area.

Your initial touch of the trigger point will likely be very tender to your dog. Monitor your animal's feedback and keep reassuring him with a soft voice. After 10 to 20 seconds, the tenderness will decrease considerably.

When dealing with an acute trigger point, you should hold a light pressure, 2 to 5 pounds, for most of the application only raising the pressure slightly to a maximum of 10 pounds at the end when you feel the trigger point releasing.

When dealing with a silent trigger point you may consider progressively raising your pressure to 15 pounds depending on the muscular mass you are working on and on the dog's reaction. When treating a trigger point in the brachiocephalicus muscle of the neck, for example, you may consider squeezing or pinching the trigger point between your thumb and index finger. Use the same pressure and duration as you would in any other situation.

Do not use more pressure than necessary; trigger points can be overtreated. The ideal pressure is the one which gives a sensation somewhere between pleasure and pain. Evaluate the pressure applied relative to your dog's feedback; watch the eyes. You may apply a continuous pressure or consider alternating pressures (for example, light to heavier, back to light, 2 or 3 times). If the pressure is too heavy, the dog will certainly let you know. Play it safe!

Once released, trigger point areas should be drained thoroughly with plenty of effleurages. Then, to further the treatment, use light frictions along the length of the whole muscle fiber - or the whole muscle bundle - in which the trigger point was located. This along with the effleurage will increase the drainage. Drainage after trigger point

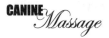

release is most important. As you break down a long-standing build-up of toxins, you must move those toxins into the circulation in order to avoid creating a worse condition. Drainage will also bring fresh blood, new oxygen and nutrients to greatly assist the healing process.

The area where the trigger point(s) was located may be very sore for a few hours, or even a day or so, due to the inflammation of the nerve endings. In that case wait a day or two before working deep on the same area again. In the meantime, apply light effleurages and wringings plus gentle finger frictions daily if possible to increase the blood circulation through that area and to assist recovery. If some degree of inflammation is present use cold hydrotherapy after the treatment to soothe the nerve endings and boost the circulation.

The trigger point technique is used very often as part of the maintenance routine, discussed later, and in sport massage treatments after heavy exercise or play. Lightly exercising your dog immediately after this type of work is recommended if your dog is not too inflamed and fatigued. Gentle exercise such as walking or light trotting will allow the muscles to recover their full contractile power and elasticity, flush fresh blood through the fibers and will maximize the effect of the treatment.

Stress Point Technique

The stress point technique is used to release stress points. Stress points are microspasms involving only a few fibers out of a whole bundle of fibers. However, these microspasms can turn into full-blown muscle spasms. If a stress point is not inflamed it is referred to as a "dormant" stress

point. If a stress point is inflamed it is referred to as an "active" stress point which will display more tenderness and will eventually produce heat and swelling. Many dogs experience tight muscles resulting in reduced muscle action such as a shorter stride or lameness due to stress point development within these muscles.

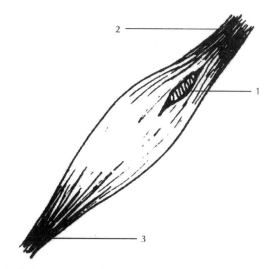

6.4 Schematic Diagram of a Stress Point

(1) stress point, usually found by the origin tendon
(2) origin tendon
(3) insertion tendon

How Stress Points Form

Stress points form as a result of great mechanical stress which causes micro-tearing of the muscle fibers. Heavy training, repetitive actions, weight overload, strenuous effort and so on are all examples of great mechanical stress.

Stress points also develop as a response to trauma such as a bump, a fall or as a result of overstretching. After an injury and during the recovery stage, the muscular compensation developing in the rest of a dog's body will trigger formation of other stress points within the compensatory muscles. For example, a dog with a sore carpus may develop compensatory stress points in the shoulder muscles as well as in the muscle attaching the scapula to the rest of the body. If really lame, the dog will switch his weight onto the other legs to relieve pressure on the sore carpus causing a great deal of muscular strain on the other limbs and resulting in new stress point formation.

It is important to remember that the inflammation process—the body's natural healing response to any trauma—can lead to a vicious circle of pain, tension, inflammation, more pain and so on. The inflammation process could therefore result in the formation of more stress points. A bad case of a sore back or hip is a good example of this phenomenon. Keep the inflammation under control by using hydrotherapy to cool the area and maintain the inflammation at a "healthy" level. Use lots of effleurages to ensure proper flow of blood to the area which brings in fresh oxygen and nutrients.

Where Stress Points Form

Stress points can be found anywhere in the muscular structure of the dog. Due to the nature of the dog's locomotor system, there are some well-known areas of the skeleton and related specific muscles where stress points are usually found. More detailed information on the location, diagnosis and treatment of stress points can be found in Chapter 8.

Stress points will most often develop at a muscle's tendon of origin. The tendon of origin is the tendon that anchors the muscle to the stable,

non-movable body part during a concentric contraction. The tendon of origin tends to be quite strong and of good size because it is the anchor attachment for the muscle and therefore sustains great mechanical strain. The other tendon, the tendon of insertion, attaches the muscle to the movable part. This tendon is not as strong or as large as the tendon of origin but will sometimes show stress, especially during isometric contractions to stabilize the body and eccentric contractions when absorbing great tension during landing, for example.

The dog, like humans, works all of its body at once. Muscle tightening does not remain in an isolated area. It transmits from one muscle to another, from one muscle group to another. As one group tightens up, the antagonist group must compensate for the loss of movement and therefore experiences extra stress. You may find several stress points during a treatment. Some are related, some are not.

How Stress Points Feel

A stress point feels like a spot of hardened, rigid tissue about the size of the end of your little finger or less. It does not move under the fingers, may be slightly swollen and it will feel tender to the dog when touched. Also a tight line of muscle fibers within the muscle bundle associated with the stress point will be felt across the muscle.

During an acute stage or an inflammation flair-up, stress points will show up very quickly. They are easily detectable because of their tenderness and of the presence of heat and swelling. If the stress point area appears inflamed, use cold hydrotherapy to numb the nerve endings prior to your treatment. Apply the swelling technique if nec-

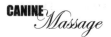

essary and follow with the stress point technique. When inflammation is present, work very lightly progressing gently into deeper massage over a few sessions to relieve the inflammation.

During chronic stages, the stress points will be more difficult to detect because the symptoms of heat and swelling are less evident. But with practice, you will develop a feel for stress points and will recognize them easily. If no inflammation is present, you may consider using heat or vascular flush over the area to loosen the fibers prior to your treatment.

When Stress Points Form

Stress points can form at any time, especially when the dog is under a lot of strain, is fatigued by intense playing or training, or when there is chronic pain from an old injury or a chronic condition such as arthritis. Older dogs show arthritic deterioration in leg joints where the consequent pain causes muscle tension. This muscle tension triggers more arthritic degeneration in the joints. Massage can help break this cycle of muscle tension and stress point build-up. Not to forget that stress points will sometimes appear in response to a direct trauma.

How Dogs Respond To Stress Point Work

The animal's response to your work will vary greatly with the degree of inflammation present in the muscle tissue. With stress points, the pain reaction you get in relation to your pressure indicates the severity of the stress. To assess the stress point, start with a light pressure which you then progressively build up.

From experience in human therapy practice, pain caused by a stress point is not normally as sharp as that in a trigger point but it can be severe on occasion and especially during acute inflammation. The initial contact on the stress point may elicit some tenderness but soon a feeling of relief will replace the original discomfort.

When a stress point is "dormant" or non-active, mild pressure from 8 to 12 pounds applied to it will cause a skin twitching reaction. After a few minutes, a general "let go" of the muscle worked on will occur. Most often dogs seem to enjoy this form of work.

When a stress point is "active" or inflamed the reaction will be more pronounced. As you apply light pressure to an active stress point, you will notice excessive skin twitching and flinching; the animal will pull away from the pressure. If the reaction is sharp or if the adjacent muscles are showing excessive tightness, you may suspect that the muscle may be close to full spasm. Be very gentle and methodical in your approach.

Stress Point Technique Outline

The stress point technique consists of two stages. One deals with the "Golgi apparatus" nerve cell, the other deals with the "muscle spindle" nerve cell. As you locate a stress point, identify the muscle it belongs to.

The Golgi

A thorough massage of the tendon of origin, with pressure applied towards the bone, will stretch the sensory nerve endings — the Golgi nerve cell — located in the tendons. While being stretched, the Golgi nerve cell will send nerve impulses to the brain and cause a reflex through the nervous system. The reflex will relax the corresponding motor nerve which is responsible for this stress point. The nervous reflex may take from a few seconds to a few minutes to occur. Small stress points may release very quickly while more chronic stress points may take several minutes. Do not overwork them.

If the stress point area appears inflamed, use cold hydrotherapy to numb the nerve endings. Otherwise, if the area does not appear inflamed, consider using heat or vascular flush over the area to loosen the fibers.

Start your technique with the SEW approach to warm up the area. Proceed with a thorough kneading massage over the tendon of origin where you have located the stress point. Then with your thumb or fingertips apply a gentle pressure of 2 or 3 pounds on the stress point to establish the initial contact and evaluate the degree of inflammation. Apply your pressure on the stress point and towards the bone where the muscle anchors. Progressively increase your pressure to 5 pounds then up to 10 to 15 pounds as the stress point release occurs.

Observe your dog's reaction as you proceed and adjust accordingly. Hold the pressure until you feel the stress point let go. Follow with lots of effleurages to thoroughly drain the area. If after a minute no release has happened, progressively release your pressure, intersperse with a few effleurages, and repeat the procedure of applying pressure to the stress point for another minute or until it releases.

The Muscle Spindle

The second stage of this technique consists of working the muscle spindle nerve cell. Use the one-hand or double-hand friction back and forth across the length of the muscle bundle to gently work the muscle spindle nerve ending. Move your fingertips very gently and perpendicularly to the grain of the muscle fibers all along their course. Using a medium pressure of eight to 12 pounds, intersperse your gentle frictions with effleurages every 20 seconds to drain the area. This will reset nerve awareness and will fully relax the muscle. Also, this gentle frictioning will loosen the tight fibers, increase circulation through the muscle, restore free motion to the fibers and decrease painful symptoms. Be aware that if you friction the muscle spindle too vigorously or with too much pressure (15 to 20 pounds) it will stretch the muscle spindle and will cause the muscle to react by contracting. Be gentle during this phase of the technique.

Follow up with the WES approach to bring in new blood, nutrients and oxygen to the site. The muscle will feel better immediately. The dog should be lightly exercised (walk-trot) immediately after the massage. When the dog is warm, use stretching exercises (see Chapter 9) to further the "let go" of the affected muscle groups.

The stress point technique is very efficient when properly applied. If under-worked, a stress point will still present the same symptoms with very little or no improvement. If you do not feel any improvement after working on a stress point for two or three minutes, stop. Overworking the tissues will aggravate the inflammation, especially in chronic tension cases; it sometimes takes several treatments to relieve a stress point.

If inflammation is present, use the ice-cup technique discussed in Chapter 10 after your treatment to cool the nerve endings and elicit vasodilation. Give the animal a couple of days of rest before further massage in that area. Keep records of your work and of the results produced. Regular practice will allow you to experiment and gain expertise.

The Origin - Insertion Technique

The origin-insertion technique will release muscle contracture and full muscle spasms, as well as strengthen muscle weakness. The origin-insertion technique is simply the stress point technique applied to both the tendon of origin and of insertion of a muscle.

"Origin-insertion" refers to the tendon of origin and of insertion of a muscle. The origin tendon is the muscle part that anchors to the most stable, least movable bone, whereas the insertion tendon attaches the muscle to the movable part, so that during contraction the insertion is brought closer to the origin. The tendon of origin is usually stronger and bigger than the tendon of insertion because its anchor attachment sustains greater stress. This stress is responsible for most of the problems found close to the tendons of origin.

Contracture can be found anywhere in the belly of the muscle. Contracture is a hypertonic state in which muscle fibers can not let go their contractile power. Many motor nerve impulses resulting from high stress, pain and inflammation cause the muscle fibers to contract indefinitely. Contractures are responsible for the decrease of muscle action which results in congestion, a lack of fluid circulation in the muscle fibers, as well as restricted movement, for example a shorter stride.

By thoroughly massaging the tendons of origin and the insertion ("Golgi sensory" nerve endings) and the whole muscle bundle ("muscle spindle" nerve endings), the origin-insertion technique will send relaxation impulses to the brain. In response,

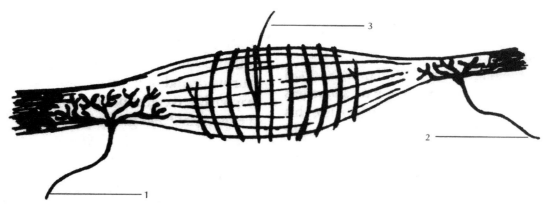

6.5 The Origin-Insertion Technique

(1) Golgi sensory nerve cell by the origin tendon
(2) Golgi sensory nerve cell by the insertion tendon
(3) Muscle spindle sensory nerve cell by the muscle bundle

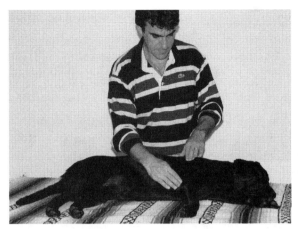

6.6 The Origin-Insertion Technique
Performed here on the triceps muscle.

the corresponding motor nerve signal causing the muscle to remain contracted will cease, releasing the spasm. This release may occur quickly or not depending on the stress level, the severity of the spasm, and whether the spasm is associated with a trauma or with a wound. Sometimes a spasm will let go only several hours after the treatment.

To derive the maximum benefit from this technique, you need a thorough knowledge of the muscle group you are working on. Knowing where the muscles attach and their direction is most important to the effectiveness of the treatment.

When dealing with a full spasm, remember that your dog is feeling a lot of pain from this condition. Use cold hydrotherapy to numb the pain and lots of strokings to comfort your animal before you start applying the origin-insertion technique.

The Origin-Insertion Technique Outline

After you locate the problem and ascertain which muscle you need to work on, begin with the SEW approach to gently warm up the muscle tissues.

Then use a gentle but firm double-thumb kneading over the tendon of origin, pressing it against the bone away from the belly of the muscle. Apply pressure at approximately 5 to 10 pounds, 15 to 20 on large muscle groups, for approximately two minutes. Intersperse with some effleurages every 20-30 seconds.

When finished on the tendon of origin, thoroughly drain the area you worked on with several effleurages. Then repeat the kneading and effleurage procedure in the same fashion on the tendon of insertion.

Next, drain the entire muscle area with thorough effleurages. Then, using your fingertips, gently friction the entire muscle at cross-fibers, back and forth. Repeat 2 or 3 times along the entire muscle length. Finish with the WES approach to ensure a thorough drainage.

Depending on the spasm's severity and the degree of inflammation present in the tissue, the origin-insertion technique should not continue for more than 10 to 12 minutes. Avoid overworking the area for this can aggravate the situation. It is better to repeat the treatment several times over a few days rather than risk irritating the nerve endings or worsening the inflammation in the muscle fibers during the first treatment.

In most acute stages, the contracture or spasm will release shortly after the first treatment - within 30 minutes or a few hours.

If the contracture is in a chronic stage, it may take several treatments to produce a positive result. In the case of a torn muscle, the origin-insertion technique is contra-indicated in the acute stage and only applied in a very gentle way in the sub-acute phase.

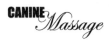

When using this origin-insertion technique to strengthen a weak muscle, you need to reverse the direction of your kneading pressure by pressing towards the belly of the muscle instead of towards the bone. This manual "stretching" of the "Golgi nerve" will result in a tonifying reaction onto the muscle. When working a weak muscle, you only need to apply this technique for about 5 to 10 minutes at a time proportional to the muscle size. Repeating the treatment several times over a few days will show tremendous improvements.

In all cases, follow with the appropriate stretch, but only if there are no torn muscle fibers!

Cold hydrotherapy is beneficial before and after treatment. Cold hydrotherapy reduces nerve irritability and cools down the inflammation.

The vasoconstriction followed by the vasodilation reaction will flush the muscle and provide more blood with new nutrients and oxygen. Heat would be more appropriate when dealing with a weak muscle.

The origin-insertion technique is used regularly in maintenance and preventive massages to stimulate and strengthen both over-exercised muscles and weak muscles.

The various techniques presented here will sharpen your skills. They will ensure the best results in maintaining your dog's fitness or assisting its recovery. These techniques will make your work more specialized, more effective and much more fun.

Massage Routines

CHAPTER 7

A massage routine is designed to provide the best results in the shortest time frame. A massage routine is a series of moves or techniques arranged in a specific order to achieve a desired result in the shortest time. A few examples are the relaxation, maintenance and recuperation routines which were created to address particular situations in the most effective way possible. These routines will contribute to the maintenance and preventive care of your animal while simultaneously giving you feedback on its general health and training level.

When a dog is restless, scared, or after a long journey, a relaxation routine will ease him fairly quickly. For the exercising dog, the maintenance routine will keep the muscular structure free from trigger and stress points, improve your dog's performance as well as making him feel good. When your dog has been training heavily, the recuperation routine will help shorten the recovery time and prevent the tightening up and stiffening of the locomotor structures. The warm up and cool down routines will assist the animal just before and after exercising. The "trouble spot" routine will help prevent muscular problems in the heavily exercised dog.

To ensure proper maintenance, most routines should be applied on a regular basis. Such a schedule will give you frequent feedback on the physical and emotional condition of your animal while contributing to the preventive aspect of your training program. Applying these routines regularly will not only develop your dog's confidence during your work, but will also encourage the animal to become deeply relaxed and trusting, thus fully responding to your massage.

The relaxation routine can be applied at any time. It is mainly used for an initial contact with the animal, before and after traveling, when putting it to rest, before a show, after a fright, and so on. When done in a shorter version, the relaxation routine can be used to start any form of massage treatment.

If the dog is in an average training program, the maintenance routines should be done regularly once or twice a week. If the dog is participating in a demanding competitive program, maintenance routines should be used on a daily basis.

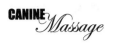

The recuperation routine should be given after every heavy training session. When a heavy training program ends, apply this routine daily for a few days until the transition to a slower pace program is complete.

Massage routines should be considered regular practice for the good health of your animal. To ensure the effectiveness of these routines, it is best to work on the dog in a quiet location, free from distractions and noise.

With practice you will become familiar with the routines outlined in this chapter. The types of movement, the rhythm and the pressure are particular to each routine; they are selected and placed in specific sequences to ensure specific results. Always start working with a gentle approach progressively increasing your pressure and rhythm when needed.

You will be able to add your own touches and eventually create your own routines according to your aims and the conditions you are treating. Trust your own judgment and be creative. But at the beginning, for safety and effectiveness, follow the guidelines given here. These routines are designed for healthy animals. If abnormal problems arise or there is strong indication of an inflammation, check with a veterinarian or registered massage therapist before proceeding.

The Relaxation Massage Routine

Dogs, like humans, experience stresses of different kinds ranging from the physical (exercises, training schedules, workload) to the emotional (abuse, boredom, lack of love or kindness, anxiety, fear). When a dog is stressed, his body will show tension, but the original stress itself is in the brain. The purpose of the relaxation routine is to relax the animal and relieve stress in a quick and efficient way. The relaxation massage routine concentrates on the nervous system only, using mostly pure nervous reflex massage moves over the spinal column from the neck, the back, the sacrum and the tail to elicit a parasympathetic nervous response.

The relaxation routine requires very little pressure and the rhythm of your movements should be very smooth, about one move per second on average. This routine will achieve positive results over the course of one to several treatments. It may put your dog to sleep, but it will also induce great relaxation and a strong relief of nervous stress. The relaxation achieved will clear nervous tension and blockages and regenerate the flow of vital energy through the spine to the rest of the body.

The relaxation routine is very effective in inducing deep relaxation at once and is good to use when approaching a dog for its first massage. It will induce great relaxation and a strong relief of the nervous system – it might even put your dog to sleep. Your dog will feel an overall improvement as a result of this routine. Even dogs of strong character will soften drastically after several relaxing massage sessions, becoming more enjoyable companions.

The Relaxation Massage Routine Outline

Use this routine when starting any other routine or massage treatment. The relaxation massage routine can also be applied before and after traveling, before, during and after competition, in the event of a scare, and if the animal has become

7.1 Relaxation Massage Routine Outline

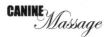

restless from boredom. When giving an animal its first massage, employ this routine, including the head massage routine, to give it a complete feeling of relaxation.

Before beginning the routine, it is important to stand beside the dog for a few minutes to connect with him. Spend a few moments gently stroking the dog's neck and the base of the ears.

1 - Poll Work (Back of the Head)

Start with three clockwise then twelve counter-clockwise gentle small circular movements with the fingertips, just behind the ears to connect with the animal for a few seconds. To reinforce the relaxed atmosphere, talk to him quietly. Then, with your right hand, massage the top of the crest of the neck with light muscle squeezing, two or three pounds pressure at the most, starting directly behind the poll and over a few inches. Apply 20 to 30 gentle muscle squeezings to trigger the parasympathetic nervous response which allows relaxation. The dog will probably lower its head as a response to your work.

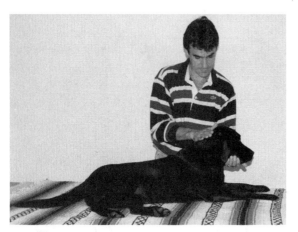

7.2 Poll Work: *Relaxation Routine*

2 - Ear Work

Gently pull the ears from the base to the tips stretching them sideways. Then gently and very lightly rub the tips between your fingers for a few seconds. This will soothe the dog. If your dog does not like his ears being worked, skip this part and spend more time massaging the crest of the neck behind the head.

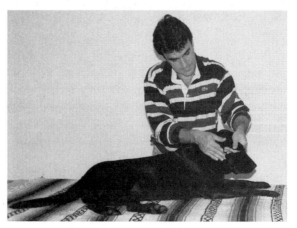

7.3 Ear Work: *Relaxation Routine*

3 - Neck Work

With one or both hands, use the muscle squeezing move along the whole upper aspect of the neck from the base of the skull down to the shoulders in one pass. Your pressure should be firm but no heavier than 5 to 8 pounds, and your rhythm smooth and slow with one muscle squeeze per 2 seconds. This particular approach will have a very soothing effect on the animal. Most dogs lower their heads willingly in this sequence and you may want to repeat with a second pass to reinforce this relaxation feeling.

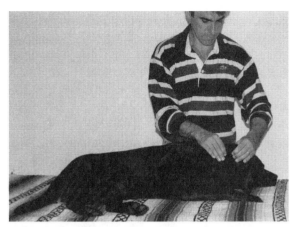

7.4 Neck Crest Work: *Relaxation Routine*

4 - Neck Rocking

This is for large dogs with very tense or thickly muscled necks; smaller animals would probably not enjoy this movement. Use some stroking moves over the entire neck in the direction of the hair in a very gentle manner. Then employ some very gentle neck rocking movements to further relax the whole neck. To do so, place one hand on the upper aspect of the neck and your other hand on the windpipe for support, then gently rock the top of the neck back and forth. Build up slowly

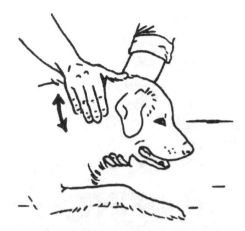

7.6 Neck Rocking Movement: *Relaxation Routine*

to a rhythm of one movement per second. Start at the upper neck and slowly, over 6 to 8 rocking motions, go down to the shoulders. This will greatly loosen the large muscle group of the neck.

5 - Upper Shoulder Work

After the neck rocking, stroke the neck downward and start to massage the whole upper shoulder area on both sides with very smooth muscle squeezing. Be gentle throughout. Use 3 to

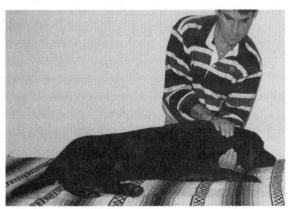

7.5 Neck Rocking Movement: *Relaxation Routine*

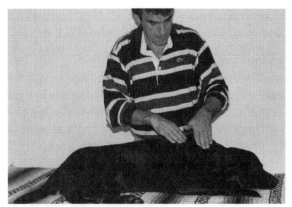

7.7 Upper Shoulder Work: *Relaxation Routine*

5 pounds pressure for approximately 1 minute. Intersperse with light strokings every 30 seconds for 3 to 5 seconds at a time.

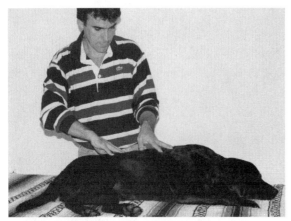

7.8 Back Work: *Relaxation Routine*

6 - Back Work

Follow with 2 or 3 light long strokes over the entire back. Keep the pressure very light at 1 or 2 pounds maximum and the rhythm very smooth.

7 - Sacrum Work

As you finish your back work, place your right hand over the sacrum bone. Hold it there with a light vibration for 10 to 30 seconds. Then make 3

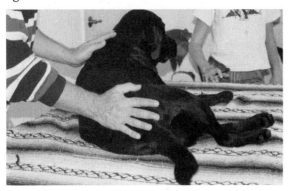

7.9 Sacrum Work: *Relaxation Routine*

slow clockwise circular motions, reversing to anti-clockwise motions for 15 to 20 circles. This particular move will strongly stimulate the parasympathetic nervous response.

8 - Tail Work

After the sacrum work, switch your right hand with your left hand to keep contact with the dog. With the right hand, use gentle point pressure along the tail bone, then the rump and flow to the next move. Pick up the tail with your right hand; take the tail a few inches from its base, bringing it upward. Use your left hand as well to stretch the tail into a question mark.

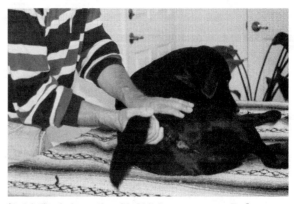

7.10 Raising the Tail Movement: *Relaxation Routine*

Gently move the tail in a circle, 3 times clockwise and 3 times anti-clockwise. Take note of any movement restriction on either side of the tail; this is a sign of muscle tension in the tail muscles and the hindquarters.

At this point, move yourself to the rear of the dog and pull on his tail very gently. Hold this stretch for approximately 30 seconds to a minute unless the dog shows signs of discomfort. Usually the

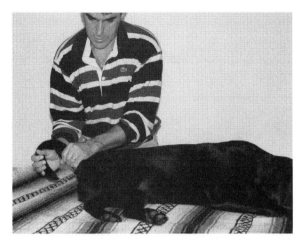

7.11 Question Mark Movement: *Relaxation Routine*

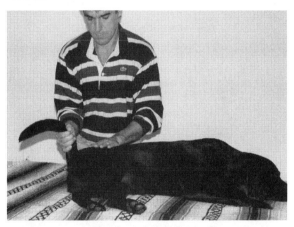

7.12 Turning Tail Movement: *Relaxation Routine*

dog responds positively by pulling against your traction. Stretching the tail will contribute to and increase the dog's relaxation tremendously.

While stretching the tail with one hand, use the other hand's thumb and fingers to gently work each vertebra from the base of the tail downward with a few muscle squeezings. Reverse the hands if you prefer.

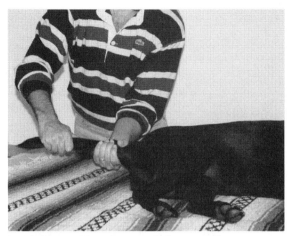

7.13 Stretching the Tail Out: *Relaxation Routine*

Take note of the tail's flexibility, any tender spots or points of possible inflammation. Release the tail stretch progressively and then stroke the hind quarters and sacrum area for a few seconds.

9 - Leg Work

After the tail work, proceed with a gentle stroking down the legs. Never lose the hand contact. Use 2 to 3 strokings on the way down the leg and 2 or 3 on the way up, adding a few more over the upper body as you move from leg to leg. Since

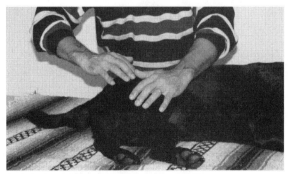

7.14 Stroking the Hind Legs Down: *Relaxation Routine*

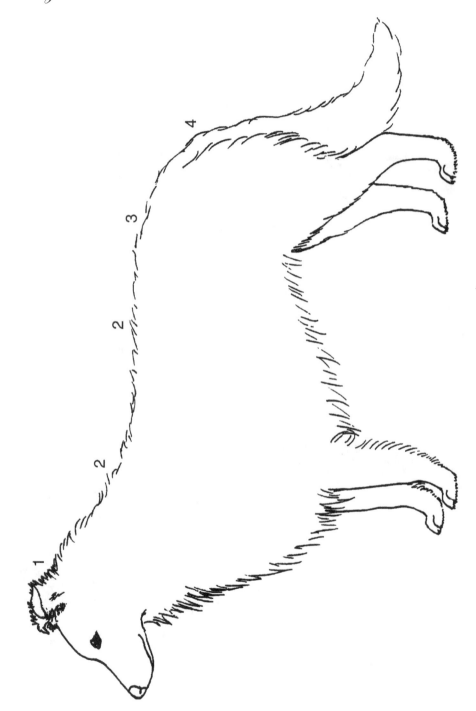

7.15 Relaxation Massage Routine Short Version Outline

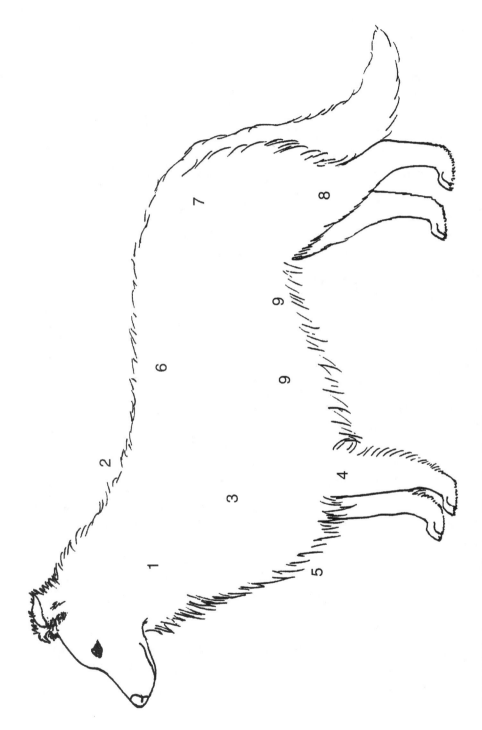

7.16 Maintenance Massage Routine Outline

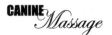

you are already at the rear, start with the hind legs. Then, with a few stroking movements, move to the front legs, a repeat the same approach on the front legs.

Pick up each leg in a gentle manner. Then when the leg is flexed, move it gently in a small circle inwards, then forward, to the outside, then back. Start again, repeating the movement 2 or 3 times. This action will further the relaxation and the let-go feeling in the legs and indirectly over the rest of the body. Be gentle! This relaxation routine should take from 10 to 15 minutes depending on the dog's size. You can take longer if you want, but the point of this routine is to initiate the relaxation reflex in a short time frame. Ten minutes is ideal.

Short Version of the Relaxation Routine

When you use the relaxation routine as a starter before another routine, a shorter version of the relaxation routine can be used. Skip the muscle squeezings over the crest of the neck, the neck rocking, the upper shoulder work, and the leg work at the end. Perform the routine movements in the following order:

1. Start with circular movements right behind the upper neck

2. Use strokings down the neck, over the back, all the way to the sacrum.

3. Work the sacrum.

4. Work the tail as described above. When finished with the tail, flow back to the neck using strokings and go on to the other routine or technique.

In the early stage of connecting with the dog, it is highly recommended that you use the full relaxation routine until the animal gets used to the relaxation associated with this particular massage routine. Experience shows that this routine outline works very well. It won't take long before the dog associates his relaxation with your work. So with practice, you will be surprised how quickly your dog will feel relaxed.

The Maintenance Massage Routine

This routine is intended to keep the muscular and skeletal structure fit, to assist circulation of body fluids and to remove toxins. The maintenance massage routine also gives you a chance to evaluate and massage all muscle conditions (tension, knots, stress points and trigger points) and to detect any other abnormal symptoms. At any time in the maintenance routine, you can add appropriate techniques to deal with particular situations such as swellings, stress points, trigger points. If any abnormal problems should arise, please check with your veterinarian before proceeding with your massage.

Remember that on your first contact with the dog, your pressure should be light, becoming firmer as you progress into the massage.

Maintenance Massage Routine Outline

Connect with the animal for a few seconds by talking quietly and gently massaging the upper neck with light muscle squeezings.

1. Start at the base of the neck with the SEW approach covering the entire neck. Then use muscle squeezings along the top of the spine

from the ears all the way to the shoulders. With thumb or finger kneadings, thoroughly work the various neck muscles. Intersperse with effleurages every 10 seconds. Your pressure should be light at the beginning, 2 or 3 pounds, progressing to a firmer touch of 8 to 10 pounds pressure. Your overall rhythm should be smooth - 1 to 2 movements per second. Consider using gentle hand frictions to loosen the muscles. Finish by draining the neck with the WES approach.

2. Moving to the withers area, start with the SEW approach then use muscle squeezings, thumb kneadings and gentle frictions to work thoroughly all of the muscle attachments. Intersperse every 10 seconds with effleurages (5 to 8 pound pressure) and finish with the WES approach before moving to the shoulder.

3. Use the SEW approach to warm up the entire shoulder area. Then use light kneadings

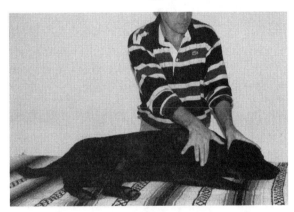

7.17 Maintenance Massage: *Upper Neck Work*

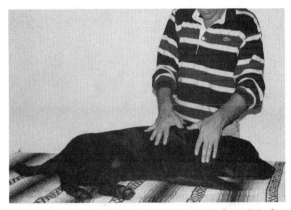

7.19 Maintenance Massage: *Withers Work*

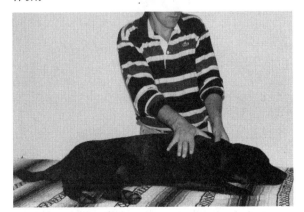

7.18 Maintenance Massage: *Neck Work*

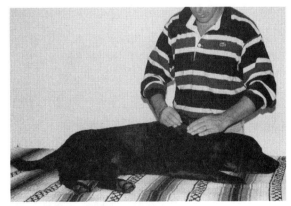

7.20 Maintenance Massage: *Lower Neck and Withers Work*

(thumbs, fingers or palms) and gentle finger frictions, interspersed with effleurages, along the muscles of the scapula. The serratus thoracis muscle often shows tension; use compression moves to loosen the fibers of this muscle, followed by gentle finger frictions. Drain the area thoroughly with the WES approach.

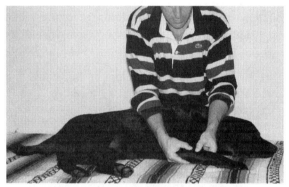

7.21 Maintenance Massage: *Foreleg Work*

4. To work the leg, begin by gently stroking down the foreleg for a grounding effect. Then, progress with the SEW approach. Starting at the point of shoulder, use muscle squeezings, picking-ups, kneadings and

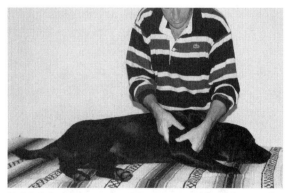

7.22 Maintenance Massage: *Shoulder Work*

gentle frictions, interspersed with effleurages, over the triceps muscle as well as the fleshy part of the flexor and extensor muscle groups. Gentle muscle squeezings, gentle frictions and thumb kneadings will loosen the tendons and stimulate the blood circulation all the way down to the paw; intersperse with effleurages going up the entire leg. Finish the leg with the WES approach.

5. Gently weave your strokings over to the front chest and complete the SEW approach over that area. Then use large kneadings, muscle squeezings, vibrations, shakings, gentle kneadings and compressions to massage the pectoral muscles and the point of the shoulder. Intersperse with effleurages every 20 to 30 seconds. Be creative. Then use the WES approach over the area and weave your strokings back over the shoulder all the way to the withers.

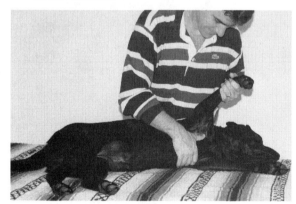

7.23 Maintenance Massage: *Chest Work*

6. Use the SEW approach over the back and up and down the spine to stir up the circulation. Follow with light tapotements on the back muscles to reach deep into the muscle

structures along the spine. Intersperse with effleurages every 30 seconds on average. Finger or palmar kneadings and light frictions will help loosen the fibres of the longissimus muscle group of the back. Finish the back with the WES approach.

Use large wringings interspersed with effleurages up and down the ribcage 2 or 3 times. Use light kneadings between the ribs and intersperse with effleurages toward the heart. You can use large shakings to stimulate the circulation over the chest area.

Do not overdo the shakings as this may be more stressful than enjoyable to the animal. You may consider using tapotement moves in the form of light (3 to 5 pounds pressure) clapping/cupping and hacking to deeply stimulate the circulation. Always follow with thorough effleurages. Also consider using the skin rolling move as it is very efficient to keep the skin and underlying fascia loose.

7. Moving to the gluteus and hamstring muscles, use the SEW approach to warm up the area. Then apply tapotements and compressions to

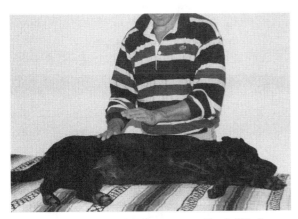

7.24 Maintenance Massage: *Back Work*

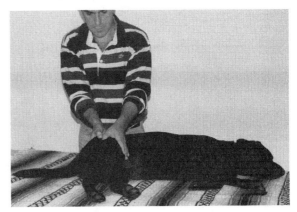

7.26 Maintenance Massage: *Gluteus Work*

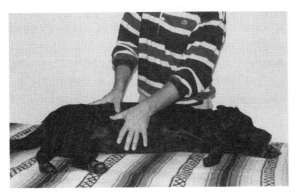

7.25 Maintenance Massage: *Ribcage Work*

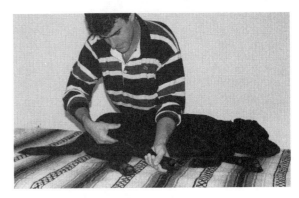

7.27 Maintenance Massage:
Hamstring Work

stir up the circulation and to loosen the fibers of this large muscle group. Use thumbs, fingers or palmar kneadings and gentle finger frictions along the length of the fibers of all the muscle groups of the hind. Intersperse with effleurages towards the stifle and finish this area with the WES approach.

8. Begin with the SEW approach on the hind legs, then effleurage upward towards the flank area. Then use gentle muscle squeezings, kneadings and gentle frictions, all interspersed with effleurages every 10 seconds over the fleshy part of the flexor and extensor mus-

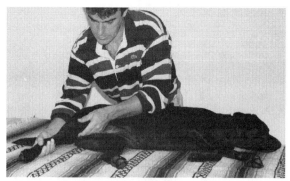

7.28 Maintenance Massage: *Hind Leg Work*

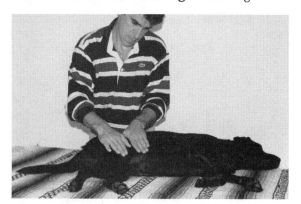

7.29 Maintenance Massage: *Hind Leg Drainage Work*

cle group of the hind leg. Drain thoroughly upward starting from the top of the leg and working your way down. Once at the bottom of the leg, effleurage from the paw to the stifle in one long stroke; repeat to cover all aspects of the limb. Gentle muscle squeezings, gentle frictions and thumb kneadings will loosen the tendons and stimulate the blood circulation to the muscle all the way down to the paw; finish the hind leg with the WES approach going up the entire leg.

9. With effleurages, flow back to the thorax area. Gently reposition your dog and repeat this sequence on the other side of his body. The overall routine can last between 20 and 30 minutes depending on your goal, the temperament of the dog and his size. Keep it on the short side when in the early stage of massaging your dog. With repetition, your dog will become more receptive to your massage work, and once he has become accustomed to it, it will not be unusual to see a maintenance massage routine last for an hour for a large dog.

The maintenance massage routine will give you feedback on the physiological state of your dog and will help you detect problems early and prevent any small ones from becoming more serious. As you find trigger points, stress points, swellings and inflammations, take notes and apply the appropriate techniques. Always follow with lots of effleurages.

The maintenance routine is a wonderful tool for maintaining and increasing the dog's performance. Regular use of the routine, at least once a week, will give you feedback on the quality of your training and will warn you of any potential problems. For highly trained dogs, this routine should be applied at least every second day.

Due to the frequency of the massage application, you will find that 20 to 30 minute sessions are sufficient to keep your dog in top shape and will prevent any serious muscular problems from hampering your dog's performance.

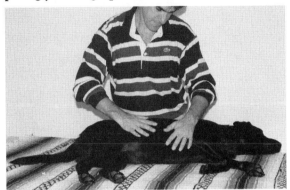

7.30 Maintenance Massage: *Thorax Drainage Work*

The Recuperation Massage Routine

The recuperation routine is a great help in avoiding the build-up of lactic acid, which is responsible for the formation of trigger points especially after heavy exercising. This routine is intended to assist the lymphatic circulation and speed up recovery time. For this purpose we will mostly use lots of effleurages, gentle wringings and large thumb or finger kneadings, depending on the area you are working on.

The recuperation routine is usually applied after exercise. Hydrotherapy (see Chapter 10) is very useful in this routine, as swollen nodes are very sore to the touch. If an inflammation is present,

use cold hydrotherapy to relieve the irritation. Otherwise, if there is no sign of inflammation, use the vascular flush or heat to relieve congestion and assist with circulation of the lymph fluid.

Lymph channels run everywhere in the body but are mostly located along the spine and the deep arteries. Lymph nodes - glands that act as filters to clean bacteria and unwanted particles - are found along the lymph channels. Lymph nodes are also found in patches at the junction of the limbs and the trunk on the inside of the legs.

The recuperation routine should be performed very gently because you are dealing with irritated tissues due to inflamed nerve endings, in response to high levels of lactic acid. Use mostly effleurage moves done lightly with 2 or 3 pounds pressure over the tender areas, 5 to 7 pounds on thicker muscle groups. When no strong inflammation is present, you may use light vibrations over specific lymph node areas; it is very effective in decongesting and stimulating the circulation. Gentle thumb, finger or palmar kneadings may be used to stir up the circulation in thick muscle areas.

Use a light 3 to 5 pound pressure around the leg joints with small, light, circular effleurages. In a recuperation routine, drain the lymphatic fluid in the direction of the heart; but first decongest swollen and inflamed nodes before bringing more fluid to them. Use cold hydrotherapy to soothe nerve endings and cool off the inflammation. If you have to deal with patches of enlarged lymph nodes, apply the swelling technique routine to decongest them. Start at the periphery of the nodes, using light circular effleurages and drain the nodes from the center towards the outside.

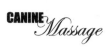

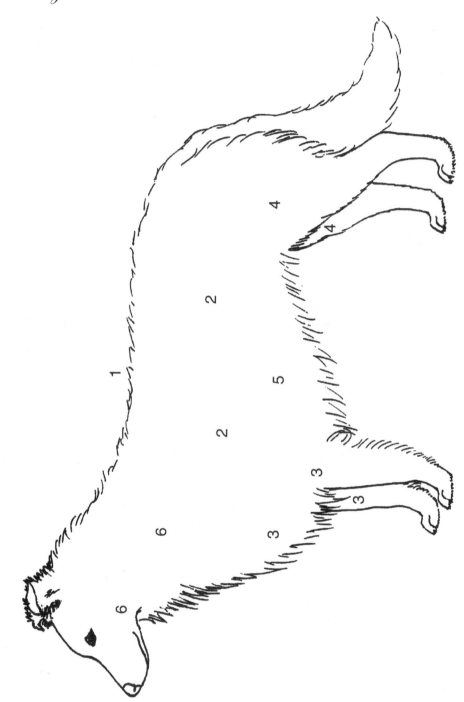

7.31 Recuperation Massage Outline

Recuperation Massage Routine Outline

Connect with the animal for a few seconds by talking quietly and apply the short version of the relaxation routine.

1. Begin the recuperation routine at the base of the neck, on the left side of the dog. Use effleurages to drain along the entire spine all the way to the croup. Repeat 2 or 3 times.

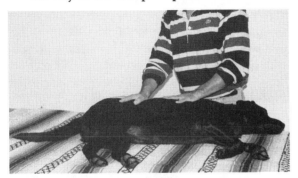

7.32 Recuperation Routine: *Effleurage of Back*

2. Position yourself halfway between the fore and hind legs of your dog. Drain the thorax area with effleurages from the spine downwards along the rib cage. Effleurage the first

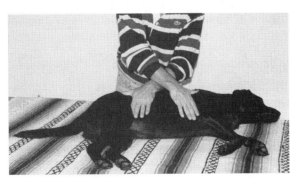

7.33 Recuperation Routine: *Effleurage of Thorax*

half of the rib cage toward the inside of the foreleg and the second half of the rib cage towards the inside of the hind leg. Repeat each aspect 2 or 3 times. Repeat this work on the other side of the dog.

3. Work the chest with lots of effleurages and kneadings, draining downward between the inside of the foreleg towards the heart. Use gentle shaking moves on the large shoulder muscles. Work the left leg by using effleurages scooping toward the inside leg. Work progressively down the leg draining it upwards. Because toxins may be found all the way down to the paw, thoroughly drain the leg up towards the heart. Repeat this work on the right leg.

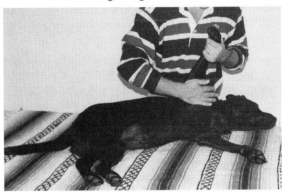

7.34 Recuperation Routine: *Inside Fore Leg Effleurage*

4. Repeat this procedure on the hind legs. Be gentle when working over the tendons of the lower legs. When working at the back of the dog, move the tail to the side in order to reach the upper attachments of the hamstring muscle groups. Scoop your effleurage movements towards the inside of the leg. If in this location the patches of lymph nodes appear

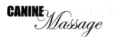

swollen and inflamed, first apply a cold towel to soothe the nerve endings and follow with a gentle swelling technique.

5. Proceed with effleurages over the dog's back, scooping downward onto the chest. Massage all the way to the neck.

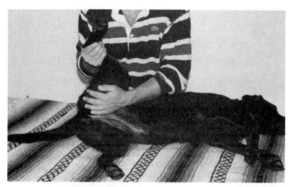

7.35 Recuperation Routine: *Inside Hind Leg Effleurage*

6. Spend some extra time draining the base of the skull and the top of the neck behind the poll thoroughly; use gentle muscle squeezings interspersed with effleurages. These moves will help drain the lymph nodes located in the upper neck. Move to the head and drain

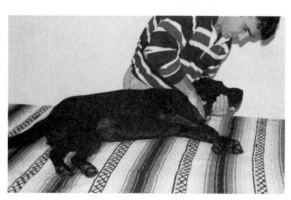

7.36 Recuperation Routine: *Neck Effleurage*

the area under the jaw along the throat latch and the trachea back towards the neck. To finish this routine and soothe the dog, use a lot of light strokings over the entire body from neck to tail and down the legs.

Remember that a dog showing stiffness and some lymphatic inflammation will be fairly sensitive. The sensory nerve endings are very tender and will therefore respond quickly to pressure. Be very gentle when you start this routine. Constantly check the feedback signs from the dog as you proceed. Pay close attention to what your fingers tell you, focusing on the 4 T's. Your starting pressure should be 1 or 2 pounds. Gently build to between 3 and 5 pounds if the dog appears comfortable. The recuperation routine should last between 15 to 20 minutes.

The Warm Up Massage Routine

This routine is designed to stimulate blood circulation in a short period of time to perk up the dog before exercising. The massage will bring more blood, oxygen and nutrients to the muscle fibers. The routine is not a replacement for warm up exercises, but it is nonetheless a valuable start.

For this routine, use mostly stimulating movements such as shakings, wringing-ups, tapotements interspersed with plenty of effleurages. Perform the routine briskly—but not to the point of irritating the dog—with movements performed at a rhythm of 2 or 3 strokes per second. Your pressure should vary from five to seven pounds in the beginning and up to 10 and 15 pounds when going over large muscle groups. Start gently progressively increasing the rhythm and pressure of your moves. Remember, the intent is to stir the blood circulation and perk up the dog, not to spend time performing deep massage on specific muscles.

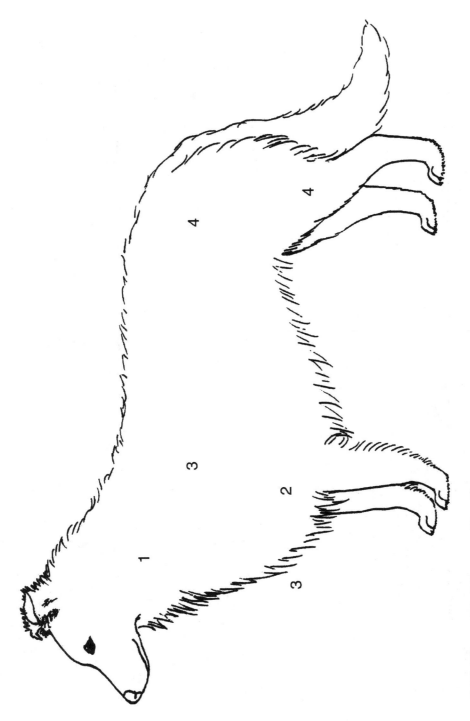

7.37 Warm Up Massage Routine

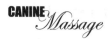
Warm Up Massage Routine Outline

Connect with the animal for a few seconds by talking quietly and gently massaging the poll and the upper neck with light muscle squeezings.

1. Begin on the left side of the neck with light shakings and use a gentle rhythm of 1 stroke per second, slowly increasing the pace to 2 or 3 strokes per second. Then switch to wringings, covering the whole neck all the way down to the left shoulder and upper leg. Thoroughly cover all muscles and intersperse with effleurages every 20 to 30 seconds as well as when moving from one body part to another.

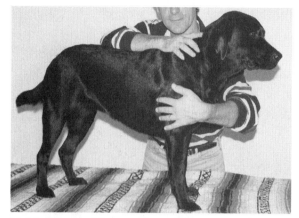

7.39 Warm Up Routine: *Upper Foreleg Shaking*

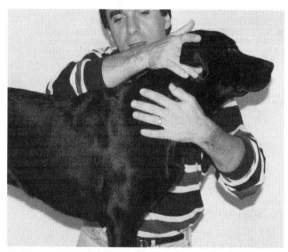

7.38 Warm Up Routine, *Fine Shaking Lower Neck*

2. Thoroughly massage the upper leg both on the inside and outside. Use shakings, wringings, picking-ups and large kneadings interspersed with effleurages. Drain towards the heart, starting from the upper leg and working down with every move. Once at the bottom of the leg, drain the entire leg with two

long effleurage strokes from the paw to the shoulder. Keep your pressure moderate and your rhythm swift.

3. Next, massage the chest thoroughly with shakings, muscle squeezings and kneadings, draining the area with effleurages every 20 or 30 seconds.

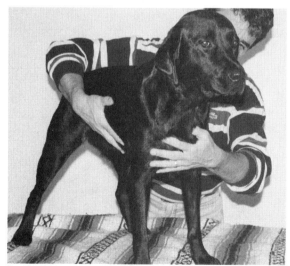

7.40 Warm Up Routine: *Chest*

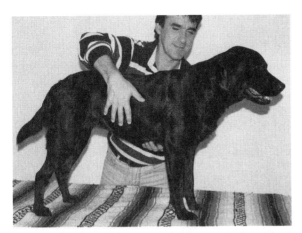

7.41 Warm Up Routine: *Thorax Shaking*

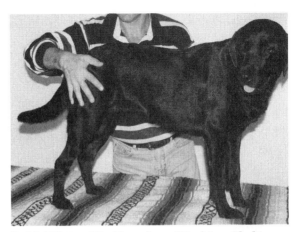

7.42 Warm Up Routine: *Hind Leg Shaking*

Go back over the shoulder with some effleurages or strokings, working your way to the withers. From there, apply wringings across the entire back, 2 or 3 times, interspersed with effleurages. Proceed with some tapotements, starting with clappings and then hackings, followed by effleurages. Using shakings, work the entire back and rib cage. Drain towards the heart with effleurages every 20 seconds as you progress. Watch for the feedback signs from the dog. You should slow down the pace as you reach the groin area, since it is a very sensitive area and dogs are naturally very protective of it.

4. Next, go over the large muscle group of the hindquarters and down to the stifle and hock, using shakings, wringings, large palmar kneadings, compressions, all interspersed with effleurages every 20 or 30 seconds. Work the hind leg in the same way as the foreleg. Start from the top, draining it upward as you work your way to the lower aspect of the limb.

Repeat the entire routine on the right side. When you have completed this, apply a gentle wringing over the back and croup followed by effleurages. Keep the routine to 10-15 minutes. Longer sessions of the warm up routine would irritate the dog. Indeed, the size of the dog is an important factor to consider: the more to massage, the longer the routine. Immediately before the exercise, apply the shaking move over the entire legs and the large muscles of the shoulder and hind quarters. This will deliver an extra last minute touch to perk up your dog.

Cool Down Massage Routine

The purpose of the cool down routine is to loosen the muscles and generate good blood circulation immediately after exercising so as to prevent stiffening and loss of flexibility. This routine should be applied as soon as the walking cool down period is finished. In application, the cool down routine is very close to the warm up routine, but here the emphasis in on drainage and the relaxation of the muscle groups by using lighter pressure and slower rhythm.

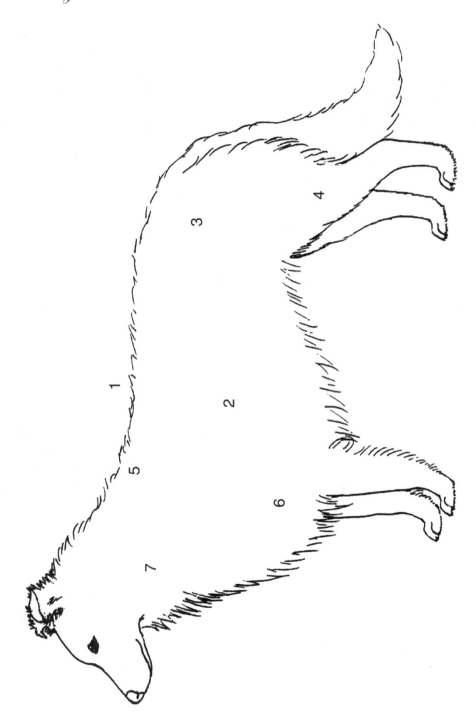

**7.43 Cool Down Massage Routine
Outline**

Cool Down Routine Outline

1. Start with generous wringings up and down the entire back, 3 to 5 times, interspersed with 15 to 20 generous effleurages. Follow with kneadings on the back muscles to relax the tendon attachments along the bones of the spine.

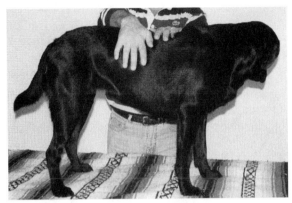

7.44 Cool Down Massage Routine:
Wringing Over Back

2. Apply larger shakings with some light hackings over the whole rib cage to clear any lactic acid from the deep muscle layers. Follow with effleurages draining towards the heart.

3. Move on to work the hind quarter with wringings, compressions, kneadings, all interspersed with effleurages.

4. Work the hind legs with large kneadings and effleurages, beginning at the upper aspect of the leg, above the stifle, effleuraging upward. Use 15 to 20 small effleurages until you reach the bottom of the leg, then from the paw, effleurage all the way up the whole leg. Repeat three or four times to cover all aspects of the leg (inside, outside, front and back). Do both legs.

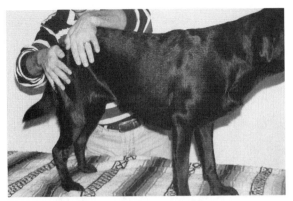

7.45 Cool Down Massage Routine:
Wringing Over Hindquarters

5. Using several effleurages or strokings, move back to the withers and apply thorough kneadings over the muscle attachments to relax them. Drain the withers thoroughly with effleurages.

6. Then move on to work the shoulders and forelegs with wringings, kneadings, picking-ups on the leg below the elbow, all interspersed with

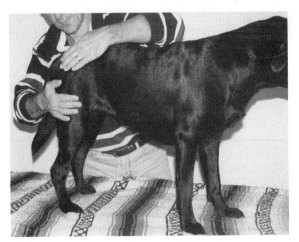

7.46 Cool Down Massage Routine:
Effleurage Hind Leg

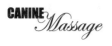
effleurages every 20 or 30 seconds. Drain the forelegs in the same manner as you drained the hind legs. When finished with the legs, use light compressions, kneadings and effleurages to work the chest muscles.

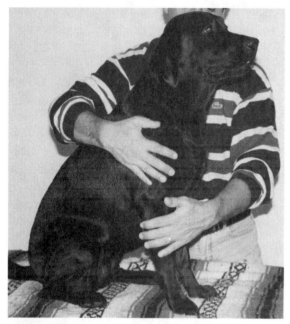

7.47 Cool Down Massage Routine:
Effleurage Forelegs

7. Finish this area with thorough wringings up and down the entire neck, followed by large kneadings and muscle squeezings over the crest of the neck. Follow with lots of effleurages.

The overall time of this routine should be under 20 minutes. It is a good idea to follow the routine with stretching exercises (see Chapter 9) to

help clear and reset the muscles after the workout and cool down routine. If during your work you detect stress or trigger points or other abnormalities, use the appropriate techniques to remedy the situation. See Chapter 8 for the trouble spot massage routine which is a nice complement to a maintenance massage routine, especially if your dog exercises regularly.

With practice you will become familiar with each routine and will discover what works best for your dog. You will even be able to create your own variations. Be innovative and try different approaches. When in doubt about the effect of a specific routine, check with your canine massage therapist.

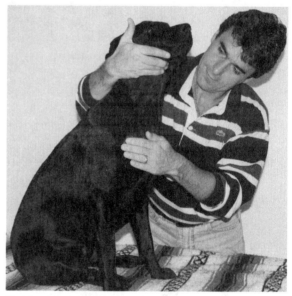

7.48 Cool Down Massage Routine:
Effleurage of Neck

Common Stress Areas

To improve the quality of your work, you need to know the most common stress areas found in the dog and their corresponding muscular stress points. Stress areas refer to those areas where several muscle groups attach. In this chapter, the following four important body "regions" will be discussed:

• The head and neck

• The shoulders and forelegs

• The back and rib cage

• The hind quarters and hind legs

During intense muscular activity, these areas will show tension of varying degree ranging from a mild tightness to chronic contracture and eventual spasm. Many dogs experience tight muscles resulting in reduced muscle action. Remember that the whole muscle structure of the dog works simultaneously, and you will most likely find more than one stress area. In the case of a recovery from injury, aside from the actual pain of the injury, you will find compensatory muscle tension in the other limbs and on the back and neck.

For each stress point you will learn:

• Its location and the motion it affects

• Its signs and symptoms

• The way it feels on palpation

• Important structures involved and massage recommendations

A thorough knowledge of these stress points will give you a better appreciation of your dog's fitness and where to apply your massage. The appropriate massage will directly affect your dog's physical performance, allowing for better muscular contraction with more power, a greater flexibility and increased overall coordination. If the stress point is well defined consider using the "origin-insertion" technique discussed in the Chapter 6.

Head and Neck

The head and neck play an important role in the dog's movements. Good flexibility of both the head and neck is vital to performance. A dog uses his head and neck constantly to balance the rest of his body. This is obvious during run-

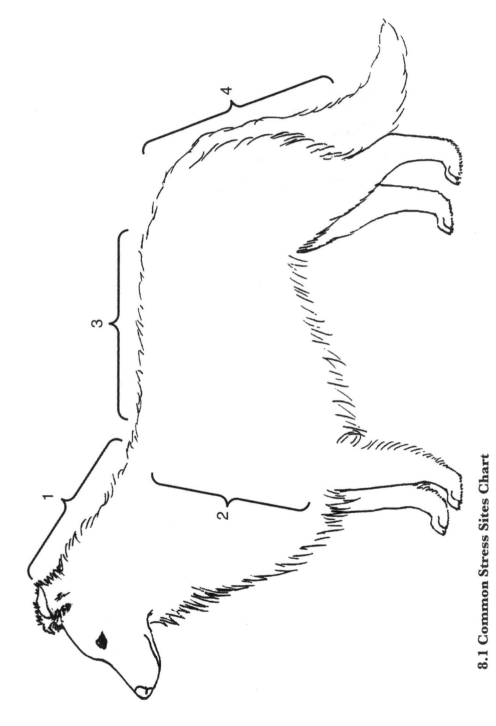

8.1 Common Stress Sites Chart

1) Head and Neck Section
2) Shoulder and Foreleg Section
3) Back and Rib Cage Section
4) Hindquarter Section

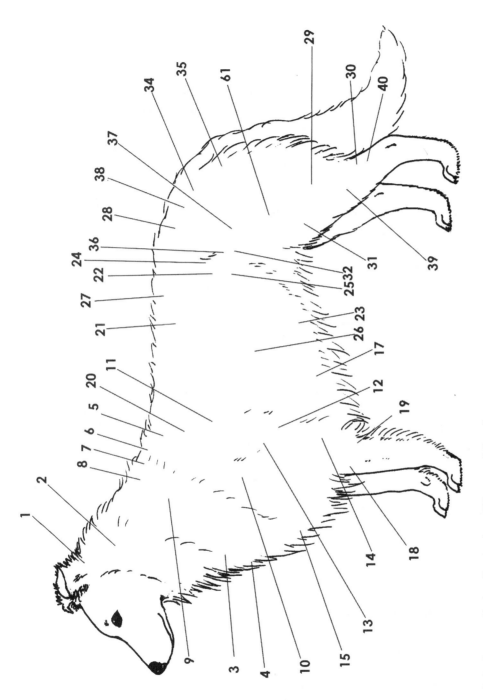

8.2 Stress Point Location Chart, side view

General Canine Stress Point Chart

1 **Sternocephalicus Muscle** - *Flexion and lateral flexion of the head*
2 **Splenius Muscle** - *Lateral flexion of the head*
3 **Cleidocephalicus Muscle** - *Sideways head and neck movement, lifts foreleg*
4 **Sternomastoideus Muscle** - *Flexes neck to the side, rotates head to opposite side*
5 **Serratus Dorsalis Cranialis Muscle** (anterior) - *Extends the back, lift ribs (inhalation)*
6, 7, 8 **Rhomboideus and Trapezius Muscles** - *Draw scapula upwards, forward and backward*
9 **Supraspinatus Muscle** - *Extension of shoulder joint, prevents dislocation*
10 **Deltoideus Muscle** - *Abduction of should joint and contributes to flexion of the foreleg*
11 **Serratus Ventralis Thoracic Muscle** - *Draws scapula backwards, draws truck upwards*
12 **Latissimus Dorsi Muscle** - *Draws leg backward*
13 **Triceps Muscle** (Proximal End) - *Flexes shoulder joint*
14 **Triceps Muscle** (Distal End) - *Extends and locks elbow joint*
15 **Superficial Pectoral Muscle** (Cranial End) - *Abducts foreleg during movement*
16 **Superficial Pectoral Muscle** (Caudal End)- *Abducts foreleg during movement*
17 **Deep Pectoral Muscle** - *Abducts and draws foreleg backwards on movement*
18 **Carpal Extensor Muscles** - *Extend paw during movement*
19 **Carpal Flexor Muscles** - *Flex paw during movement*
20 **Longissimus Dorsi Muscle** - *Extends back and loins, lateral flexion*
21 **Iliocostalis Muscle** - *Lateral flexion of the trunk*
22 **External Abdominal Oblique Muscle** (hip) - *Flexes trunk straight and laterally*
23 **Internal Abdominal Oblique Muscle** (ribcage) - *Flexes trunk straight and laterally*
24 **Internal Abdominal Oblique Muscle** (belly) - *Flexes trunk straight and laterally*
25 **Transversus Abdominus Muscle** - *Flexes trunk straight and laterally*
26 **Intercostal Muscles** - *Flex trumk straight and laterally*
27 **Junction of the Middle Gluteal & Longissimus Dorsal Muscles** - *Forward propulsion*
28 **Biceps Femoris Muscle** - *Extend and abducts hindleg, flexes stifle*
29 **Biceps Femoris Muscle** (belly part) - *Flexes stifle*
30 **Gastrocnemius Muscle** - *Etension of hock, flexion of stifle*
31 **Vastus Lateralis Muscle** - *Flexion hip/femur*
32 **Rectus Femoris Muscle** - *Flexion hip/femur*
33 **Adductor Muscles** (femur insertion) - *Adduct hind leg*
34 **Semitendinosus Muscle** - *Extends hip, flexes stifle*
35 **Semimembranosus Muscle** - *Extends hip, flexes stifle*
36 **Tensor Fasciae Latae Muscle** - *Flexes hip, rotates thigh outward*
37 **Iliopsoas Muscle** - *Flexes hip, rotates thigh outward*
38 **Superficial Gluteal Muscle** - *Extends hip*
39 **Digital Extensor Muscles** - *Extend paw during movement*
40 **Digital Flexor Muscles** - *Flex paw during movement*

8.3 Superficial Muscle Layer with Stress Point Locations

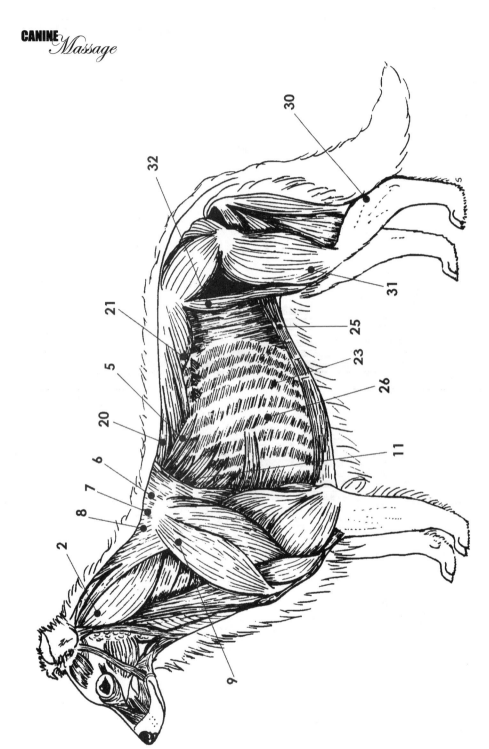

8.4 Deep Muscle Layer with Stress Point Locations

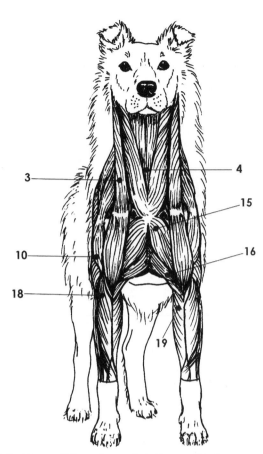

8.5 Front Muscles with Stress Point Locations

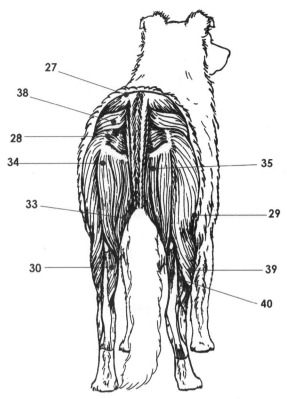

8.6 Back Muscles with Stress Point Locations

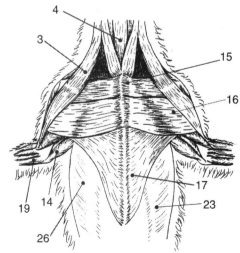

8.7 Ventral Muscles with Stress Point Locations

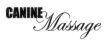

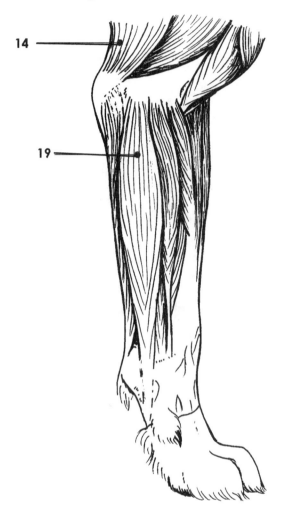

14

19

8.8a Foreleg Muscles with Stress Point Locations (medial view)

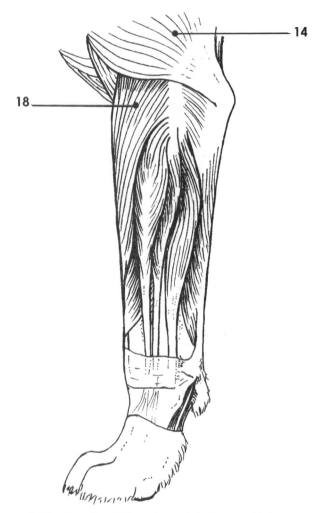

14

18

8.8b Foreleg Muscles with Stress Point Locations (lateral view)

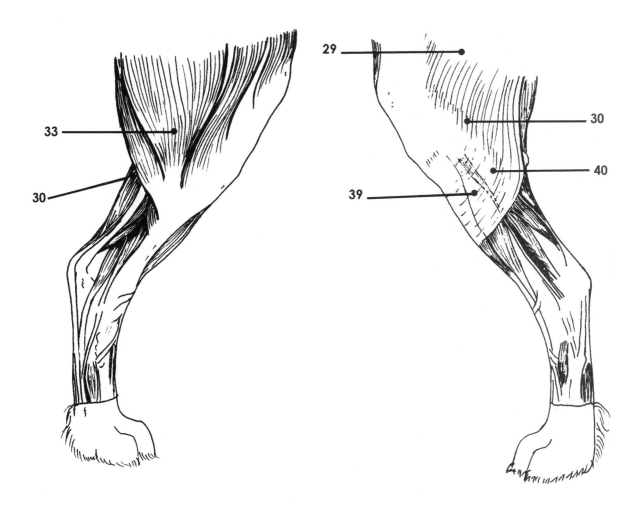

8.9a Hindleg Muscles with Stress Point Locations (medial view)

8.9b Hindleg Muscles with Stress Point Locations (lateral view)

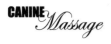

ning—the downward swing of the head will help lift the rear legs off the ground as the dog moves forward. The head and neck are also very active when the dog plays, for example when catching a stick, a Frisbee or a ball. Especially when a dog plays "tug of war", a tremendous amount of strain is put on the entire musculoskeletal system of the neck as well as the rest of the body.

1. The Sternocephalicus Muscle: *Muscle Flexion and Lateral Flexion of the Head*

Located in the superficial layer, this muscle is found on each side of the neck attaching to the mastoid process of the temporal bone of the skull, running downward to anchor on the sternum. When it contracts bilaterally, it flexes the head. When it contracts unilaterally it moves the head laterally, on the side of the contraction.

When this muscle is tight, the dog shows discomfort, pulling the head to that side, resisting sideways motion to the opposite side. At rest, the dog will have a tendency to keep his head flexed to the tight side, and during motion he will clearly show head discomfort.

SP 1 is located close to the tendon of insertion by the temporal bone, the spinous process of the second cervical vertebrae and the nuchal ligament. It may feel very tender to the dog. When you apply pressure to SP 1, the dog will drop his head. If the point is very tender to the dog he will flinch and perhaps try to pull away from the pressure. This is a sign of excessive tightness and stress; if you feel heat under your fingers, suspect inflammation. The muscle will feel tight along its entire course, proportional to the severity of the muscular stress. If the stress point is well defined, consider also working the tendon of origin by the sternum using the "origin-insertion" technique.

2. The Splenius Muscle: *Lateral Flexion of the Head*

Located in the deep layer, this muscle is found on each side of the neck attaching to the skull and running downward to anchor on the spinous processes of the first few thoracic vertebrae. When it contracts bilaterally, it extends the head. When it contracts unilaterally it moves the head laterally, on the side of the contraction.

When this muscle is tight, the dog shows discomfort, pulling the head to that side, resisting sideways motion to the opposite side. At rest, the dog will have a tendency to keep his head flexed to the tight side, and during motion he will clearly show head discomfort, showing restriction in lowering his head.

SP 2 is located close to the tendon of insertion near the transverse processes of the first three cervical vertebrae and the nuchal ligament. It may feel very tender to the dog. When you apply pressure to SP 2, the dog will lower his neck. If the point is very tender to the dog he will flinch and perhaps try to pull away from the pressure. This is a sign of excessive tightness and stress; if you feel heat under your fingers, suspect inflammation. The muscle will feel tight along its entire course, proportional to the severity of the muscular stress. If the stress point is well defined, consider also working the tendon of origin using the "origin-insertion" technique.

3. The Cleidocephalicus Muscle: *Sideways Head and Neck Movement, Lifts Foreleg*

Located in the superficial layer this muscle is found on each side of the neck attaching to the upper neck on the first five cervical vertebrae and the nuchal ligament, running downward to anchor on the tendinous band in front of the point of shoulder. When it contracts bilaterally, it flexes the head. When it contracts unilaterally it moves the head laterally, on the side of the contraction.

When this muscle is tight, the dog shows discomfort, pulling the head to that side, resisting sideways motion to the opposite side. At rest, the dog will have a tendency to keep his head flexed to the tight side, and during motion he will clearly show head discomfort, showing restriction by lowering his head.

SP 3 is located close to the tendon of insertion by the clavicular band. It may feel very tender to the dog. When you apply pressure to SP 3, the dog will lower his neck. If the point is very tender to the dog he will flinch and perhaps try to pull away from the pressure. This is a sign of excessive tightness and stress; if you feel heat under your fingers, suspect inflammation. The muscle will feel tight along its entire course, proportional to the severity of the muscular stress. If the stress point is well defined, consider also working the insertion tendon using the "origin-insertion" technique.

4. The Sternomastoideus Muscle: *Flexes Neck to the Side, Rotates Head to Opposite Side*

Located in the superficial layer, this muscle is found on each side of the neck attaching to the mastoid part of temporal bone and nuchal crest of occipital bone, running downward to anchor on the sternum. When it contracts bilaterally, it flexes the head bringing the neck down. When it contracts unilaterally it contributes to the rotation of the head and moves the head laterally, on the side of the contraction.

When this muscle is tight, the dog shows discomfort, pulling the head to that side, resisting sideways motion to the opposite side. At rest, the dog will have a tendency to keep his head flexed to the tight side, and during motion he will clearly show head discomfort, showing restriction by lowering his head.

SP 4 is located close to the tendon of origin by the sternum. It may feel very tender to the dog. When you apply pressure to SP 4, the dog will lower his neck. If the point is very tender to the dog he will flinch and perhaps try to pull away from the pressure. This is a sign of excessive tightness and stress; if you feel heat under your fingers, suspect inflammation. The muscle will feel tight along its entire course, proportional to the severity of the muscular stress. If the stress point is well defined, consider also working the insertion tendon using the "origin-insertion" technique.

Remember that all the muscles work together at once to deliver smooth action movement. With a typical active dog, most neck tension will be found in the extensor muscles (the semispinalis capitis, splenius, rhomboideus and trapezius muscles) found directly behind the back of the head and also in front of the top of shoulders. When there is tension present in these muscles, the dog may show discomfort by stretching his head downwards. When these muscles are tight, the dog may resist downward motion as well as movement to either side.

Upon palpation, you will feel both muscle attachments at the base of the skull and in front of the withers, feeling very tense, almost rigid. Sometimes, as a result of the discomfort felt by the dog, compensatory tension will build up in the flexor muscles of the neck (the cleidocephalicus, cleidobrachialis and sternocephalicus muscles). Tension in these muscles will be felt along the entire flexor group and in front of the point of shoulder. The dog will try to stretch its neck by moving its head in the opposite direction of the tension, up and to one side.

Some activities that could cause stress in the neck and head area are ball chasing, squirrel chasing, guard dog training, obedience, pulling a harness/cart/sled, agility dog training, tracking, guide work for the visually impaired, Frisbee and flyball competition, as well as the hard pulling when playing "tug of war."

Other Tension Areas in the Neck

The nuchal ligament (ligamentum nuchae): Running from the poll to the withers, it provides a strong attachment support for many the neck muscles. Muscle squeezing and gentle double hand frictions applied along its length will do wonders to relax this ligament.

The serratus ventralis cervicis: Found on both sides of the neck, this muscle attaches on the serrated medial surface of the scapula and runs forward to attach on the lower cervical spine. Its contraction causes the scapula to depress, supporting the trunk, and the lower neck to elevate.

The Omotransversarius: Found on both sides of the neck, this muscle attaches on the spine of the scapula and runs forward to attach on the atlas. Its contraction causes the scapula to move forward during the protraction of the foreleg.

The Cleidobrachialis: Found on both sides of the chest, this muscle originates on the clavicular band and runs downward to attach on the medial

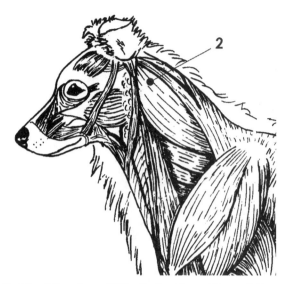

8.10a Head and Neck Section (Deep Muscle Layer) with Associated Stress Point Location

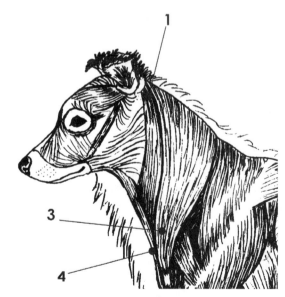

8.10b Head and Neck Section (Superficial Muscle Layer) with Associated Stress Point Locations

aspect of the humerus. Its contraction causes the humerus to move forward during the protraction of the foreleg.

The scalenus: Found on both sides of the neck, this muscle attaches along the ventral aspect of the lower cervical vertebrae and runs downward to attach to the first four ribs. When contracting together they assist the flexion of the lower aspect of the neck. The contraction of one side of the muscle will cause the neck to laterally flex and rotate turn to the same side.

The intervertebral muscles: These small muscles run on each side of the vertebral column and attach on every second vertebra. Their contraction causes the neck to rotate on itself (torque) as well as assisting lateral flexion of the neck. Stretching of the neck muscles will help bring these deep muscles into relaxation.

The Shoulder and Foreleg

A strong flexible shoulder and foreleg is essential for proper athletic performance. Good muscle power at the shoulder joint will ensure a high level of performance. This is well demonstrated during jumping as the dog uses its shoulder and stretches its leg up in front of its body during the jumping.

You may find tension in the latissimus dorsi and triceps muscles and eventually in the biceps brachii. Depending on the intensity of the workout, some tension can be found in the omotransversarius muscles that move the scapula back and forth, the supraspinatus and infraspinatus muscles of the scapula, as well as the rhomboideus, deltoideus and posterior trapezius muscles. The flexor and extensor muscle of the lower leg often show some muscle tension.

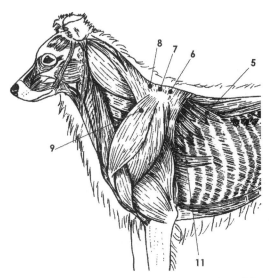

8.11a Shoulder and Foreleg Section (Deep Muscle Layer) with Associated Stress Point Locations

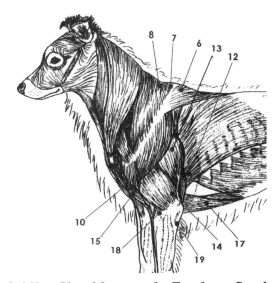

8.11b Shoulder and Foreleg Section (Superficial Muscle Layer) with Associated Stress Point Locations

The scapula has no direct joint linkage with the dog's trunk. The scapula is attached by a muscular sling that supports the thorax and reduces concussion from the front legs. The slope of the scapula and the angle formed by its junction with the humerus provides shock absorption and has much to do with the smoothness of gait we like to see during agility competitions. The scapula is pulled backward by the latissimus dorsi (SP 12) and forward by the omotransversarius muscle. The upper scapula is linked to the withers by the rhomboideus muscle, the trapezius muscle (SP 6 to 8). The deltoideus (SP 10) runs between the scapula and the humerus. The scapular spine bisects the length of the scapula, separating the supraspinatus muscle (SP 9) and the infraspinatus. These last three muscles secure the shoulder joint laterally.

The humerus moves forward when pulled by the cleidobrachialis muscle and the biceps muscle, and moves backwards when pulled by the triceps (SP 13, 14) and deltoideus and the latissimus dorsi. The deep pectoral muscle (SP 15 to 17) assists in flexion as well as providing adduction motion. Good flexibility and muscle power at the shoulder joint will ensure a high level of performance from the forelegs during running and jumping.

5. The Serratus Dorsalis Cranialis Muscle (anterior): *Muscle Extends the Back*
Located in the deep layer, this muscle is found on each side of the thoracic spine attaching to the spinous processes of the first few thoracic vertebrae (withers) and upper ribs attachment. It runs backwards and down to the side of the dog to anchor on the lower ribs. When it contracts bilaterally, it lifts the ribs during inhalation and it con-

tributes to the spinal extension. When it contracts unilaterally it contributes to lateral flexion of the dog's body.

When this muscle is tight, the dog shows discomfort upon palpation over the withers. During motion the dog will resist moving his head down and will resist lateral movement to the side opposite to the tightness.

SP 5 is felt as a deep rigid knot, located close to the tendon of insertion by the sixth thoracic vertebra. It may feel very tender to the dog. When you apply pressure to SP 5, the dog will lower his neck. If the point is very tender you might see some skin twitching along the back muscles and upper shoulders; the dog might flinch and perhaps try to pull away from the pressure. This is a sign of excessive tightness and stress. If you feel heat under your fingers, suspect inflammation. The muscle will feel tight along its entire course, proportional to the severity of the muscular stress. If the stress point is well defined, consider also working the tendon of origin using the "origin-insertion" technique.

6, 7, 8. The Rhomboideus and Trapezius Muscles: *Draw Scapula Upwards, Forward and Backward*
The trapezius (superficial layer) and the rhomboideus (deep layer) muscles share some origin attachments. Their tendons of origin anchor on the lower cervical and upper thoracic vertebrae (withers area) as well as the nuchal ligament. The rhomboideus runs down to attach along the medial dorsal border of the scapula. The trapezius runs down to attach laterally along the scapular spine. Both muscles draw the scapula upwards. The rhomboideus pulls the scapula against the trunk. The trapezius abducts the limb.

Besides being involved in the motion of the scapula, they act in concert as strong stabilizers for the foreleg, and that is the reason why they share common stress point location.

When these muscles are tight, the dog will loose some degree of flexibility. This will result in restricted motion in his foreleg movements, poor coordination and some loss of power. The withers area will be sore upon palpation. All this will trigger compensating stress point to form in other muscle group including neck, shoulders, back and hindquarters muscles.

SP 6, 7 and 8 are felt as tight lines running from withers to scapula, which will feel very tender to the dog. When you apply pressure to SP 6, 7 & 8, the dog will lower his neck. If these points are very tender to a light touch, you are dealing with the trapezius muscle. If the stress points only react to a deeper pressure, then you are dealing with the rhomboideus muscle. You might see some skin twitching along the back or neck muscles and down the shoulders; the dog might flinch and perhaps try to pull away from the pressure. This is a sign of excessive tightness and stress; if you feel heat under your fingers, suspect inflammation. Both muscles will feel tight all along their course, proportional to the severity of the muscular stress. If the stress point is well defined, consider also working the tendon of insertion using the "origin-insertion" technique.

9. The Supraspinatus Muscle: *Extension of Shoulder Joint, Prevent Dislocation*

Located in the deep layer, this muscle anchors on the anterior (or cranial) part of the scapula and attaches on the anterior aspect of the greater tubercle of the humerus. The supraspinatus and infraspinatus muscles play an important role in prevention of lateral dislocation of the shoulder joint. Any lateral work will put stress on these muscles. When contracting, the supraspinatus muscle extends the shoulder joint as well as preventing lateral dislocation.

When this muscle is tight, the dog shows discomfort with the leg on the same side. Due to the referred pain in the shoulder joint, the dog will hold its leg bent at the carpus. During motion the tightness causes lameness in the shoulder joint, resulting in abnormal stride of the foreleg in all planes, therefore affecting the dog's gait.

SP 9 is felt as a deep rigid knot by the tendon of origin in the upper end of the muscle in the upper third of the scapula. It may feel very tender to the dog. When you apply pressure to SP 9, the dog will respond by flexing is leg. If the point is very tender you might see some skin twitching along the shoulder muscles; the dog might flinch and perhaps try to pull away from the pressure. This is a sign of excessive tightness and stress; if you feel heat under your fingers, suspect inflammation. The whole muscle will feel tight all along its course, proportional to the severity of the muscular stress. If the stress point is well defined, consider also working the tendon of insertion using the "origin-insertion" technique.

10. The Deltoideus Muscle: *Abduction of Shoulder Joint and Contributes to Flexion of the Foreleg*

Located in the superficial layer, this muscle originates on the posterior aspect of the scapular spine and runs down to anchor on the deltoid tuberosity of the humerus. When it contracts, it contributes to flexion of the foreleg. This muscle also greatly contributes to stabilizing the shoulder joint in any movement.

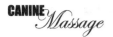

When this muscle is tight, the dog shows discomfort upon palpation over the scapula. During motion the dog will show restriction during the flexion of the shoulder causing a restricted gait. It will also resist side movements.

SP 10 is felt as a deep rigid knot, located close to the tendon of insertion by the deltoid tuberosity of the humerus. It may feel very tender to the dog. When you apply pressure to SP 10, the dog will flex his leg. If the point is very tender you might see some skin twitching along the leg muscles. The dog might flinch and perhaps try to pull away from the pressure. This is a sign of excessive tightness and stress; if you feel heat under your fingers, suspect inflammation. The whole muscle will feel tight all along its course, proportional to the severity of the muscular stress. If the stress point is well defined, consider also working the tendon of origin using the "origin-insertion" technique.

11. The Serratus Ventralis Thoracic Muscle: *Draws Scapula Backward, Draws Trunk Upwards*

Located in the deep layer, this muscle attaches on the lateral aspect of the first eight ribs and runs forward and upward to attach on the medial and dorsal aspect of the scapula. Its contraction helps to support the trunk to its proper level, and to depress the scapula.

When this muscle is tight, during motion the tightness causes lameness on the side it appears. The regular stride will be stilted on that side, interfering with the flexibility of the shoulder. The dog shows discomfort upon palpation behind the scapula by flexing his leg.

SP 11 is felt as a large tight knot, located close to the upper posterior edge of the scapula. It may feel very tender to the dog. When you apply pressure to SP 11, the dog will flex his leg. If the point is very tender you might see some skin twitching along the leg and back muscles. The dog might flinch and perhaps try to pull away from the pressure. This is a sign of excessive tightness and stress; if you feel heat under your fingers, suspect inflammation. The whole muscle will feel tight all along its course, proportional to the severity of the muscular stress. If the stress point is well defined, consider also working the tendon of origin using the "origin-insertion" technique.

12. The Latissimus Dorsi Muscle: *Draws Leg Backward*

Located in the superficial layer, this muscle originates on the thoracic and lumbar spinous processes and runs cranioventrally on each side to attach on the proximal medial aspect of the humerus of the foreleg. Its contraction is one of the main sources of power for the retraction of the foreleg. It also contributes to the medial rotation of the foreleg.

When this muscle is tight, during motion the tightness causes restriction during protraction movement on the same side it appears. The regular stride will be shortened on that side and the retraction power will be reduced. The dog shows discomfort upon palpation.

SP 12 is felt as a large tight knot by the lower aspect of the muscle close to the edge of the triceps muscle. It may feel very tender to the dog. When you apply pressure to SP 12, the dog will bring his leg backward. If the point is very tender you might see some skin twitching along the leg and back muscles. The dog might flinch and perhaps try to pull away from the pressure. This is a sign of excessive tightness and stress; if you feel heat under your fingers, suspect inflammation. The whole muscle will feel tight all along its course, proportional to the severity of the muscular stress. If the stress point is well defined, consider also working the tendon of origin using the "origin-insertion" technique.

13. The Triceps Muscle (Proximal End): *Flexes Shoulder Joint*

Located in the superficial layer, this muscle attaches on the posterior edge of the scapula and run downward to attach on the humerus and point of the elbow. Its contraction causes the shoulder joint to flex. It also extends the elbow joint.

When this muscle is tight, the dog will stand with his leg bent at the elbow and will not put weight on it while at rest. During motion, the regular stride will be shortened on that side and the retraction power will be reduced. The dog shows discomfort upon palpation of the muscle.

SP 13 is felt as a tight knot by the middle posterior edge of the scapula. It may feel very tender to the dog. When you apply pressure to SP 13, the dog will flex his leg. If the point is very tender you might see some skin twitching along the leg and back muscles. The dog might flinch and perhaps try to pull away from the pressure. This is a sign of excessive tightness and stress; if you feel heat under your fingers, suspect inflammation. The whole muscle will feel tight all along its course, proportional to the severity of the muscular stress. If the stress point is well defined, consider also working the tendon of insertion using the "origin-insertion" technique.

14. The Triceps Muscle (Distal End): *Extends and Locks Elbow Joint*

Located in the superficial layer, this muscle attaches on the posterior edge of the scapula and run downward to attach on the humerus and point of the elbow. Its contraction causes the shoulder joint to flex. It also extends the elbow joint.

When this muscle is tight, the dog will stand with his leg bent at the elbow and will not put weight on it while at rest. During motion, the regular stride will be shortened on that side and the retraction power will be reduced. The dog shows discomfort upon palpation of the muscle.

SP 14 is felt as a tight knot by the point of elbow. It may feel very tender to the dog. When you apply pressure to SP 14, the dog will flex his leg. If the point is very tender you might see some skin twitching along the leg and shoulder muscles. The dog might flinch and perhaps try to pull away from the pressure. This is a sign of excessive tightness and stress; if you feel heat under your fingers, suspect inflammation. The whole muscle will feel tight all along its course depending on the severity of the muscular stress. If the stress point is well defined, consider also working the tendon of origin using the "origin-insertion" technique.

15. The Superficial Pectoral Muscle (Cranial End): *Adducts Foreleg During Movement*

Located in the superficial layer, this muscle originates on the cranial aspect of the sternum and runs laterally to attach on the anterior aspect of the crest of humerus. Its contraction causes adduction of the foreleg. It also stabilizes the foreleg during any other motion.

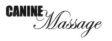

When this muscle is tight, the dog will stand on his opposite leg with his affected leg bent at the elbow and will not put weight on it while at rest. During motion, the regular stride will be somewhat shortened on that side. The retraction power will be reduced and the dog will resist abduction (lateral) movement. The dog will show discomfort upon palpation.

SP 15 is felt as a tight knot by the anterior aspect of the sternum. It may feel very tender to the dog. When you apply pressure to SP 15, the dog will adduct and flex his leg. If the point is very tender you might see some skin twitching along the leg and neck muscles. The dog might flinch and perhaps try to pull away from the pressure. This is a sign of excessive tightness and stress; if you feel heat under your fingers, suspect inflammation. The whole muscle will feel tight along its course, proportionally to the severity of the muscular stress. If the stress point is well defined, consider also working the tendon of insertion using the "origin-insertion" technique.

16. The Superficial Pectoral Muscle (Caudal End)
Adducts Foreleg During Movement
Located in the superficial layer, this muscle originates on the cranial aspect of the sternum and runs laterally to attach on the anterior aspect of the crest of humerus. Its contraction causes adduction of the foreleg. It also stabilizes the foreleg during any other motion.

When this muscle is tight, the dog will stand on his opposite leg with his affected leg bent at the elbow and will not put weight on it while at rest. During motion, the regular stride will be somewhat shortened on that side. The retraction power will be reduced and the dog will resist abduction (lateral) movement. The dog will show discomfort upon palpation.

SP 16 is felt as a tight knot before its attachment on the medial aspect of the crest of the humerus. It may feel very tender to the dog. When you apply pressure to SP 16, the dog will adduct and flex his leg. If the point is very tender you might see some skin twitching along the leg and neck muscles. The dog might flinch and perhaps try to pull away from the pressure. This is a sign of excessive tightness and stress; if you feel heat under your fingers, suspect inflammation. The whole muscle will feel tight all along its course, proportionally to the severity of the muscular stress. If the stress point is well defined, consider also working the tendon of origin using the "origin-insertion" technique.

17. The Deep Pectoral Muscle: *Adducts and Draws Foreleg Backwards on Movement*
Located in the superficial layer, this muscle originates on the sternum. It runs laterally to attach on the caudal aspect of the crest of the humerus. Its contraction, when the limb is advanced and fixed, causes the trunk to pull cranially and the shoulder to extend. When the limb is not supporting weight, its contraction pulls the limb caudally and flexes the shoulder joint. It also stabilizes the foreleg during any other motion.

When this muscle is tight, the dog will stand on his opposite leg with his affected leg bent at the elbow and will not put weight on it while at rest. During motion, the regular stride will be somewhat shortened on that side. The retraction and retraction power will be reduced. The dog shows discomfort upon palpation of the muscle.

SP 17 is felt as a tight knot by the origin tendon over the sternum. It may feel very tender to the dog. When you apply pressure to SP 17, the dog will adduct and flex his leg. If the point is very tender you might see some skin twitching along the leg and chest muscles. The dog might flinch and perhaps try to pull away from the pressure. This is a sign of excessive tightness and stress; if you feel heat under your fingers, suspect inflammation. The whole muscle will feel tight all along its course, proportionally to the severity of the muscular stress. If the stress point is well defined, consider also working the tendon of insertion using the "origin-insertion" technique.

18. The Carpal Extensor Muscles: *Extend Paw During Movement*

Located in the superficial layer, this muscle originates on the distal end of the humerus. They run distally to attach on the anterior aspect of the carpal bones. Their contraction causes the carpus joint and metacarpal bones to extend (dorsi flex).

When these muscles are tight, they will limit the protraction of the foreleg during motion, the regular stride will be somewhat shortened on that side. The dog shows discomfort upon palpation of these muscles.

SP 18 is felt as a tight knot by the origin on the humerus. It may feel very tender to the dog. When you apply pressure to SP 18, the dog might flinch and perhaps try to pull away from the pressure. If the point is very tender you might see some skin twitching along the leg and shoulder muscles. This is a sign of excessive tightness and stress; if you feel heat under your fingers, suspect inflammation. The whole muscle will feel tight along its course, proportionally to the severity of the muscular stress. If the stress point is well defined, consider also working the tendon of insertion using the "origin-insertion" technique.

19. The Carpal Flexor Muscles: *Flex Paw During Movement*

Located in the superficial layer, this muscle originates on the distal humerus and the proximal end of the ulna. They run distally to attach on the posterior aspect of the carpal and metacarpal bones. Their contraction causes the carpus to flex.

When these muscles are tight, they will limit the flexion of the foreleg during motion, the regular stride will be somewhat shortened on that side. The dog shows discomfort upon palpation of these muscle.

SP 19 is felt as a tight knot near the point of origin on the humerus and the ulna, on the medial aspect of the foreleg. It may feel very tender to the dog. When you apply pressure to SP 19, the dog might flinch and perhaps try to pull away from the pressure. If the point is very tender you might see some skin twitching along the leg and shoulder muscles. This is a sign of excessive tightness and stress; if you feel heat under your fingers, suspect inflammation. The whole muscle will feel tight along its course, proportionally to the severity of the muscular stress. If the stress point is well defined, consider also working the tendon of insertion using the "origin-insertion" technique.

When tension is present in these shoulder and foreleg muscles, the dog loses the flexibility in his shoulder movement resulting in reduced motion, coordination and power. This will also trigger compensation tension to develop in the hind quarters. The shoulder and foreleg muscles may feel tight along their course with most of their tension at the tendon of origin. If that tension develops mostly on one side, the dog will be restricted and show a shorter stride on that side. After each training session, follow with complete stretching exercises for the foreleg. Watch for discomfort, resistance or restriction in the range of motion of that limb. Take notes! Follow with a gentle massage, emphasizing drainage. Check thoroughly all related stress points.

Some activities that could cause stress on the shoulder and foreleg are: ball chasing, squirrel chasing, guard dog training, racing, hunting, herding, pulling a harness/cart/sled, tracking, flyball competition, agility competition and guiding the visually impaired.

The Back and Rib Cage

The vertebral column and the rib cage are solid structures made up of strong bones, ligaments and muscles. The role of the vertebral column is to protect the spinal cord and to provide a solid anchor for strong muscle groups. The role of the rib cage is to protect vital organs, specifically the lungs and heart.

The muscle groups of the back include: the transversospinalis system, longissimus system, iliocostalis system and dorsalis ventralis system; they contribute to the extension of the back. The external and internal abdominaloblique, the transversus abdominus , the rectus abdominus and the intercostal muscles not only stabilize the rib cage and abdomen area during movement but also strongly contribute to the flexion of the back.

20. The Longissimus Dorsi Muscle: *Extends Back and Loins, Lateral Flexion*
Located in the deep layer, this muscle originates on the crest and medial surface of the ilium as well as the spines of the lumbar and thoracic vertebrae. It courses craniolaterally, inserting on the vertebrae, both thoracic and lumbar, and the

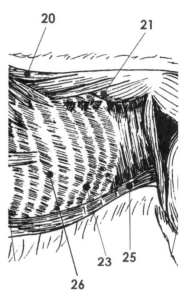

8.12a Back and Rib Cage Section (Deep Muscle Layer) with Associated Stress Point Locations

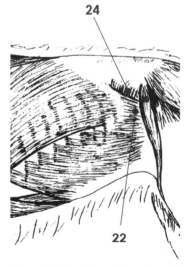

8.12b Back and Rib Cage Section (Superficial Muscle Layer) with Associated Stress Point Locations

ribs. Its bilateral contraction causes the back and loins to extend. Its unilateral contraction causes the lateral flexion of the back to the side of the unilateral flexion.

When this muscle is tight, the dog shows soreness to touch, especially when grooming. During movement the dog will be uncomfortable affecting is general flexibility during motion. The dog shows discomfort upon massage palpation of the muscle.

SP 20 is felt as a tight knot by the insertion near the withers. It may feel very tender to the dog. When you apply pressure to SP 20, the dog might flinch and perhaps try to pull away from the pressure. If the point is very tender you might see some skin twitching along the back and rib cage muscles. This is a sign of excessive tightness and stress; if you feel heat under your fingers, suspect inflammation. The whole muscle will feel tight along its course, proportionally to the severity of the muscular stress. If the stress point is well defined, consider also working the tendon of origin using the "origin-insertion" technique.

21. The Iliocostalis Muscle: *Lateral Flexion of Trunk*

Located in the deep layer, this muscle runs from C7 attaching on the ribs and continuing caudally to the point of the hip. Their contraction causes lateral flexion of the trunk and assists the extension of the back.

When these muscles are tight and pressure is put on them, the dog shows soreness. During movement the dog will show restriction in lateral bending. The dog shows discomfort upon massage palpation.

SP 21 is felt as a tight knot by the insertion on last rib. It may feel very tender to the dog. When you apply pressure to SP 21, the dog might flinch and perhaps try to pull away from the pressure. If the point is very tender you might see some skin twitching along the back and rib cage muscles. This is a sign of excessive tightness and stress; if you feel heat under your fingers, suspect inflammation. The whole muscle will feel tight along its course proportionally to the severity of the muscular stress. If the stress point is well defined, consider also working the tendon of origin using the "origin-insertion" technique.

22. The External Abdominal Oblique Muscle (hip): *Flexes Trunk Straight and Laterally*

Located in the superficial layer, this muscle originates on the tuber coxae and runs cranioventrally, inserting on the costal arch, rectus abdominus and linea alba, which inserts caudally on the symphisis pubis. Together with the internal oblique muscle, it aids in the contraction of the abdomen, flexion of the back, as well as assist lateral bending.

When this muscle is tight the dog shows restricted lateral movement during movement. The dog shows discomfort upon massage palpation of that muscle.

SP 22 is felt as a tight knot along the anterior edge of the hip bone. It may feel very tender to the dog. When you apply pressure to SP 22, the dog might flinch, perhaps try to pull away from the pressure and eventually relax his hind leg on the same side. If the point is very tender you might see some skin twitching along the back and rib cage muscles. This is a sign of excessive tightness and stress; if you feel heat under your fingers, sus-

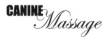

pect inflammation. The whole muscle will feel tight along its course, proportionally to the severity of the muscular stress. If the stress point is well defined, consider also working the tendon of insertion using the "origin-insertion" technique.

23. The Internal Abdominal Oblique Muscle (ribcage): *Flexes Trunk Straight and Laterally*

Located in the deep layer, this muscle originates on the tuber coxae and runs cranioventrally, inserting on the costal arch, rectus abdominus and linea alba, which inserts caudally on the symphisis pubis. Together with the external oblique muscle, it aids in the contraction of the abdomen, flexion of the back, as well as assist lateral bending.

When this muscle is tight the dog shows restricted lateral movement during movement. The dog shows discomfort upon massage palpation of that muscle.

SP 23 is felt as a tight knot in the area where the tenth rib attaches to the sternum. It may feel very tender to the dog. When you apply pressure to SP 23, the dog might flinch, perhaps try to pull away from the pressure and eventually relax his hind leg on the same side. If the point is very tender you might see some skin twitching along the back and rib cage muscles. This is a sign of excessive tightness and stress; if you feel heat under your fingers, suspect inflammation. The whole muscle will feel tight along its course, proportional to the severity of the muscular stress. If the stress point is well defined, consider also working the tendon of origin using the "origin-insertion" technique.

24. The Internal Abdominal Oblique Muscle (belly): *Flexes Trunk Straight and Laterally*

Located in the deep layer, this muscle originates on the tuber coxae and runs cranioventrally, inserting on the costal arch, rectus abdominus and linea alba, which inserts caudally on the symphisis pubis. Together with the external oblique muscle, it aids in the contraction of the abdomen, flexion of the back, as well as assist lateral bending.

When this muscle is tight the dog shows restricted lateral movement during movement. The dog shows discomfort upon massage palpation of that muscle.

SP 24 is felt as a tight thickened ridge in the middle of the muscle, an inch or two below the origin attachment. It may feel very tender to the dog. When you apply pressure to SP 24, the dog might flinch, perhaps try to pull away from the pressure and eventually relax his hind leg on the same side. If the point is very tender you might see some skin twitching along the back and rib cage muscles. This is a sign of excessive tightness and stress; if you feel heat under your fingers, suspect inflammation. The whole muscle will feel tight along its course, proportional to the severity of the muscular stress. If the stress point is well defined, consider also working the insertion tendon using the "origin-insertion" technique.

25. The Transversus Abdominus Muscle: *Flexes Trunk Straight and Laterally*

Located in the deep layer, this muscle originates from the lumbar vertebrae and medial cartilage of ribs, runs ventrally to insert on the linea alba fascia. Together with the external and internal oblique muscles, it aids in the contraction of the abdomen, flexion of the back, as well as assist lateral bending.

When this muscle is tight the dog shows general discomfort during movement and a shorter stride in the hind leg. The dog shows discomfort upon palpation of that muscle.

SP 25 is felt as a tight thickened ridge below the origin tendon and in the middle of the muscle, just about an inch in front of the point of the hip. It may feel very tender to the dog. When you apply pressure to SP 25, the dog might flinch, perhaps try to pull away from the pressure and eventually relax his hind leg on the same side. If the point is very tender you might see some skin twitching along the back and rib cage muscles. This is a sign of excessive tightness and stress; if you feel heat under your fingers, suspect inflammation. The whole muscle will feel tight along its course, proportional to the severity of the muscular stress. If the stress point is well defined, consider also working the tendon of insertion using the "origin-insertion" technique.

26. The Intercostal Muscles: *Flex Trunk Straight and Laterally*

Located in the deep layer, these muscles attach from rib to rib along the entire ribcage. Their contraction causes the thorax to compress during exhalation. These muscles can become sore from harness equipment, trauma from rough playing or accident and also from lack of exercise as seen with older animals.

When these muscles are tight the dog's breathing is shallow due to the lack of expansion of the ribcage. The dog shows discomfort upon palpation of these muscles.

SP 26 is usually felt as a tight muscle knot between the seventh and eighth ribs. This a very sensitive area and it may feel very tender to the dog. When you apply pressure to SP 26, the dog might flinch and perhaps try to pull away from the pressure. If the point is very tender you might see some skin twitching along the thorax and abdomen. This is a sign of excessive tightness and stress; if you feel heat under your fingers, suspect inflammation. The whole muscle might show tightness along the ribs, depending on the severity of the muscular stress. If the origin of the tension is due to trauma, several other intercostals muscles might show the same tightness and stress points.

When these muscles are tight due to activity, the dog will show soreness to a touch on the back and less coordinated power during motion. The dog will eventually show restriction in lateral bending of the opposite side. You may also find compensatory muscle tension in the longissimus dorsi, the semispinalis and the iliocostalis muscles. When there is lots of jumping involved, the abdominal muscles will also show tension by the hip and ribs attachments.

Some activities that could cause stress on the back and rib cage are: ball chasing, squirrel chasing, racing, flyball, herding, guard dog training, agility, hunting, tracking and pulling a harness/cart/sled. For the latter, carefully palpate the areas where the harness contacts the dog's body. Check for any inflammatory symptoms that might be present in the muscular tissues.

The Hindquarters and Pelvic Limb

The hindquarters is a very important part of the dog's anatomy as it is considered the engine of the dog. The landmarks of the hind quarter that can be palpated are: point of croup (wing of the ilium), point of buttock (ischial tuberosity), point of the hip (greater trochanter of the femur) and stifle joint (femur, tibia and patella).

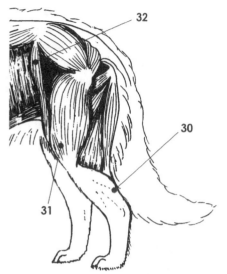

8.13a Hindquarter Section (Deep Muscle Layer) with Associated Stress Point Locations

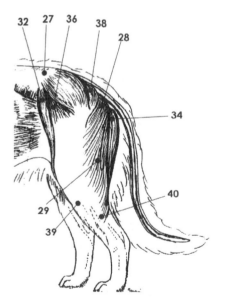

8.13b Hindquarter Section (Superficial Muscle Layer) with Associated Stress Point Locations

The conformation of the hind quarters and hind legs will determine the dog's performance ability in a given activity. The longer legs and the more angle at the joint, the greater the predisposition for sprinting and jumping as seen with the greyhound dogs.

The bulky muscles of the hind quarters anchor strongly to the lumbar spine and the pelvis. They run distally and attach to the femur and tibia. Some of the muscles moving the femur include iliopsoas (SP 37), the middle and deep gluteal (SP 38), the sartorius (SP 32), the quadriceps femoris (SP 31) and the tensor fascia latae (SP 36). When these muscles develop tension, the dog shows discomfort in his back with restricted hip motion and shortened leg protraction and retraction. Some of the muscles which move the tibia include the gastrocnemius (SP 30), the biceps femoris (SP 28-29), the semitendinosus (SP 34) and the semimembranosus (SP 35). When these muscles show tension, the dog may show lameness from the pelvic limb, restricted protraction, a loss of power during retraction and eventually a sore back. When the gastrocnemius gets tight, the dog will show discomfort in standing on that leg. You may also find tension along the lumbar and the sacral portions of the spine where many of the muscle groups attach.

27. The Junction of the Middle Gluteal & Longissimus Dorsi Muscles: *Forward Propulsion*

Located in the superficial layer, these muscles originate on the crest of the ilium and runs distally to attach on the greater trochanter. The longissimus dorsi muscle located in the deep layer, originates on the crest and medial surface of the ilium as well as the spines of the lumbar and thoracic vertebrae and it courses craniolaterally, inserting on the vertebrae, both thoracic and lumbar, and the ribs. Their actions are involved in motion (retraction).

When these muscles are tight the dog is uncomfortable when standing, keeping his leg bent at the stifle when at rest. If the dog sinks down or sags when his back is touched, this is a sure sign of a sore back. The dog shows discomfort upon palpation of these muscles. You will also observe during movement that the dog will lack power of protraction, eventually showing lameness in the hind legs.

SP 27 is felt as a tight knot an inch away from the spine at the level of the point of the croup. This a very sensitive area and it may feel very tender to the dog. When you apply pressure to SP 27, the dog might flinch and perhaps try to pull away from the pressure. If the point is very tender you might see some skin twitching along the back and hindquarters. The dog might flex his hind leg on the same side during your work. This is a sign of excessive tightness and stress; if you feel heat under your fingers, suspect inflammation. Both muscles might show tightness along their course, depending on the severity of the muscular stress. If the stress point is well defined, consider also working the tendon of insertion using the "origin-insertion" technique.

28. The Biceps Femoris Muscle: *Extends and Abducts Hindleg, Flexes Stifle*

Located in the superficial layer, this muscle originates on the sacrotuberous ligament and the ischiatic tuberosity. It courses craniodistally to attach to the patella, patellar ligament and cranial border of the tibia. Its contraction causes the stifle to flex during the non weight bearing phase of

retraction and it assist the extension of the hip, stifle and tarsus during retraction. It also contributes to externally rotate the stifle during retraction. It is a major component of the hamstring group of muscles.

When this muscles is tight, the dog will hold his leg loose (flexed at the stifle) or will try to stretch the leg by tucking under the hind end. The dog shows discomfort upon palpation of these muscles. During movement, the dog will show lameness and shortened protraction.

SP 28 is felt as a tight knot an inch away from the spine, past the sacrum. This a very sensitive area and it may feel very tender to the dog. When you apply pressure to SP 28, the dog might flinch and perhaps try to pull away from the pressure. If the point is very tender you might see some skin twitching along the hindquarters and he might flex the stifle on the same side. This is a sign of excessive tightness and stress; if you feel heat under your fingers, suspect inflammation. The whole muscle might show tightness along its course, proportional to the severity of the muscular stress. If the stress point is well defined, consider also working the tendon of insertion using the "origin-insertion" technique.

29. The Biceps Femoris Muscle (belly part): *Flexes Stifle*

Located in the superficial layer, this muscle originates on the sacrotuberous ligament and the ischiatic tuberosity. It courses craniodistally to attach to the patella, patellar ligament and cranial border of the tibia. Its contraction causes the stifle to flex during the non weight bearing phase of retraction and it assist the extension of the hip, stifle and tarsus during retraction. It also contributes

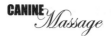
to externally rotate the stifle during retraction. It is a major component of the hamstring group of muscles.

When this muscles is tight, the dog will hold his leg loose (flexed at the stifle) or will try to stretch the leg by tucking under the hind end. The dog shows discomfort upon palpation of these muscles. During movement, the dog will show lameness and shortened protraction.

SP 29 is felt as a tight knot at the bifurcation of the muscle bundle, in the lower third of the muscle. This a very sensitive area and it may feel very tender to the dog. When you apply pressure to SP 29, the dog might flinch and perhaps try to pull away from the pressure. If the point is very tender you might see some skin twitching along the hindquarters and he might flex the stifle on the same side. This is a sign of excessive tightness and stress; if you feel heat under your fingers, suspect inflammation. The whole muscle might show tightness along its course, proportional to the severity of the muscular stress. If the stress point is well defined, consider also working the tendon of origin and insertion using the "origin-insertion" technique.

30. The Gastrocnemius Muscle:
Extension of Hock, Flexion of Stifle
Located in the deep layer, this muscle originates on the medial and lateral supracondyle tuberosities of the femur and run distally to attach to the dorsal surface of the tuber calcanei of the tarsus. Its contraction causes the stifle to flex and the tarsus to extend.

When this muscle is tight, the dog will hold his leg loose (flexed at the stifle) and will show discomfort when standing. The dog shows soreness upon palpation of this muscle. During movement, the dog will show lameness and shortened stride.

SP 30 is felt as a tight hardened bundle of fibers a couple inches above the tarsus. This a very sensitive area and it may feel very tender to the dog. When you apply pressure to SP 30, the dog might flinch and perhaps try to pull away from the pressure. If the point is very tender you might see some skin twitching along the hindquarters and he might flex the knee on the same side. This is a sign of excessive tightness and stress; if you feel heat under your fingers, suspect inflammation. The whole muscle might show tightness along its course, proportional to the severity of the muscular stress. If the stress point is well defined, consider also working the tendon of origin by the femur using the "origin-insertion" technique.

31. The Vastus Lateralis Muscle: *Flexion Hip/Femur*
Located, in the deep layer, this muscle originates on the greater trochanter and runs cranioventrally to insert on the tibial tuberosity. Its contraction causes the stifle to extend during protraction. It is a major component of the quadriceps group of muscles.

When this muscle is tight, the dog will hold his leg loose (flexed at the stifle). The dog is not comfortable standing on his leg and will show discomfort upon palpation of this muscle. During movement, the dog will show lameness and shortened protraction as well as restricted abduction.

SP 31 is felt as a tight knot above the stifle joint on the lateral aspect of the hind leg. This a very sensitive area and it may feel very tender to the dog. When you apply pressure to SP 31, the dog might flinch and perhaps try to retract the leg away from the pressure. If the point is very tender you might see some skin twitching along the hindquarters and he might flex the knee (stifle) on the same side. This is a sign of excessive tightness and stress; if you feel heat under your fingers, suspect inflammation. The whole muscle might show tightness along its course, proportional to the severity of the muscular stress. If the stress point is well defined, consider also working the tendon of origin using the "origin-insertion" technique.

32. The Rectus Femoris Muscle: *Flexion Hip/Femur*

Located in the deep layer, this muscle originates on the ilium and runs craniodistally to insert on the tibial tuberosity. Its contraction causes the stifle to extend during protraction. It is a major component of the quadriceps group of muscles.

When this muscles is tight, the dog will hold his leg loose (flexed at the stifle) and will be uncomfortable standing. He will show discomfort upon massage palpation of this muscle. During movement, the dog will show lameness and shortened protraction.

SP 32 is felt as a tight muscle knot an inch below its origin tendon. This a very sensitive area and it may feel very tender to the dog. When you apply pressure to SP 32, the dog might flinch and perhaps try to pull away from the pressure. If the point is very tender you might see some skin twitching along the hindquarters and he might flex the knee (stifle) on the same side. This is a sign of excessive tightness and stress; if you feel heat under your fingers, suspect inflammation. The whole muscle might show tightness along its course, proportional to the severity of the muscular stress. When SP 32 is present, the tendon of insertion of the rectus femoris muscle will also show tightness. Use the "origin-insertion" technique.

33. The Adductor Muscles (femur insertion): *Adducts Hindleg*

The adductor muscles are the adductor longus, the adductor magnus and brevis. They are located in the deep layer and the gracilis muscle is located in the superficial layer. They originate on the pelvic symphysis and run distally to attach to the proximomedial femur. The gracillis inserts on the cranial tibia and the tuber calcanei. Their contraction causes the hind leg to adduct, and the hip to extend. They play an important role in stabilizing the hind leg during any movements.

When these muscles are tight, the dog will hold his leg loose (flexed at the stifle) and will uncomfortable standing. He will show discomfort upon palpation of this muscle. During movement, the dog will show lameness and a shortened protraction and retraction. He will also resist abduction of his hind leg.

SP 33 is felt as a tight muscle knot on the inside of the leg, about an inch right above the medial aspect of the knee. This a very sensitive area and it may feel very tender to the dog. When you apply pressure to SP 33, the dog might flinch and perhaps try to pull away from the pressure. If the point is very tender you might see some skin twitching along the inside of the hindquarters and he might flex the knee (stifle) on the same side. This is a sign of excessive tightness and stress; if you feel heat under your fingers, suspect inflammation. The whole muscle group might show tightness along its course, proportional to the severity of the muscular stress. If the stress point is well defined, consider also working the tendons of origin of these different muscles using the "origin-insertion" technique.

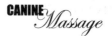

34. The Semitendinosus Muscle: *Extends Hip, Flexes Stifle*

Located in the superficial layer, this muscle originates on the ischiatic tubrosity and runs distally to attach to the medial aspect of the tibia and tuber calcanei. Its contraction causes the stifle to flex during protraction and assist extension of the hip and tarsus during retraction. It is a major component of the hamstring group of muscles.

When this muscles is tight, the dog will hold his leg loose (flexed at the stifle) and will uncomfortable standing. He might even tuck his leg under his hind end. He will show discomfort upon massage palpation of this muscle. During movement, the dog will show lameness and shortened protraction. The dog might resist forward stretching of the hind leg.

SP 34 is felt as a tight muscle knot an inch away from the origin tendon by the coccygeal vertebrae. This a very sensitive area and it may feel very tender to the dog. When you apply pressure to SP 34, the dog might flinch and perhaps try to pull away from the pressure. If the point is very tender you might see some skin twitching along the hindquarters and he might flex the knee (stifle) on the same side. This is a sign of excessive tightness and stress; if you feel heat under your fingers, suspect inflammation. The whole muscle might show tightness along its course, proportional to the severity of the muscular stress. If the stress point is well defined, consider also working the tendon of insertion using the "origin-insertion" technique.

35. The Semimembranosus Muscle: *Extends Hip, Flexes Stifle*

Located in the superficial layer, this muscle originates on the ischiatic tuberosity and runs distally to insert to the distal femur and proximal tibia.

Its contraction causes the hip to extend, assist stifle extension during retraction, and flexion during protraction and adduct the limb. It is a major component of the hamstring group of muscles.

When this muscles is tight, the dog will hold his leg loose (flexed at the stifle) and will uncomfortable standing. He might even tuck his leg under his hind end. He will show discomfort upon palpation of this muscle. During movement, the dog will show a shortened protraction as well as will track inwards. The dog might resist forward stretching as well as lateral pulling of the hind leg.

SP 35 is felt as a tight muscle knot an inch away from the origin tendon by the coccygeal vertebrae. This a very sensitive area and it may feel very tender to the dog. When you apply pressure to SP 35, the dog might flinch and perhaps try to pull away from the pressure. If the point is very tender you might see some skin twitching along the hindquarters and he might flex the knee (stifle) on the same side. This is a sign of excessive tightness and stress; if you feel heat under your fingers, suspect inflammation. The whole muscle might show tightness along its course, proportional to the severity of the muscular stress. If the stress point is well defined, consider also working the tendon of insertion using the "origin-insertion" technique.

36. The Tensor Fasciae Latae Muscle: *Extends Hip, Flexes Stifle*

Located in the superficial layer, this muscle originates on the point of the hip and runs distally to attach to the lateral femoral fascia. Its contraction causes the hip to flex and the stifle to extend.

When this muscles is tight, the dog will hold his leg loose (flexed at the stifle) and he will be uncomfortable standing, tucking his hind leg under his hind end. He will show discomfort upon massage palpation of this muscle. During movement, the dog will throw is leg outward during protraction. The dog might resist lateral movement.

SP 36 is felt as a tight muscle knot an inch away from the origin tendon by the point of the hip. This a very sensitive area and it may feel very tender to the dog. When you apply pressure to SP 36, the dog might flinch and perhaps try to pull away from the pressure. If the point is very tender you might see some skin twitching along the hindquarters and he might flex the stifle on the same side. This is a sign of excessive tightness and stress; if you feel heat under your fingers, suspect inflammation. The whole muscle might show tightness along its course, proportional to the severity of the muscular stress. If the stress point is well defined, consider also working the tendon of insertion using the "origin-insertion" technique.

37. The Iliopsoas Muscle: *Flexes Hip, Rotates Thigh Outward*

Located in the deepest layer (not shown on muscle chart), this muscle originates on the lumbar vertebrae and ventral ilium and runs caudoventrally to insert on the lesser trochanter. Its contraction causes the hip joint to flex during protraction and it assists the outward rotation of the thigh. The iliopsoas muscle is considered the primary hip flexor muscle, being responsible for the early aspect of the hind leg protraction.

When this muscles is tight, the dog will hold his leg loose (flexed at the stifle) and will uncomfortable standing. He might even tuck his leg under his hind end. He will show discomfort upon massage palpation of this muscle. During movement, the dog will show discomfort in the back and leg resulting in lameness and a shortened protraction, especially during circles on the same side. The dog might resist backward stretching of the hind leg.

SP 37 is felt as a tight line of muscle fibers all along its course. This a very sensitive area and it may feel very tender to the dog. When you apply pressure to SP 37, the dog might flinch and perhaps try to pull away from the pressure. If the point is very tender you might see some skin twitching along the back muscles and the hindquarters. This is a sign of excessive tightness and stress; if you feel heat under your fingers, suspect inflammation. The whole muscle might show tightness along its course, proportional to the severity of the muscular stress. The tendon of insertion is not palpable due to its location, making it difficult to apply the "origin-insertion" technique.

38. The Superficial Gluteal Muscle: *Extends Hip*

Located in the superficial layer, this muscle originates on the sacrum and ilium and runs distally to insert to the third trochanter. Its contraction causes the hip joint to extend during retraction and it assists abduction of the thigh.

When this muscle is tight, the dog will show discomfort in his back with restricted hip motion and shortened protraction of the hind leg. He will show discomfort upon palpation of this muscle. The dog might resist forward stretching or adduction of the hind leg.

SP 38 is felt as a rigid knot about one inch from its origin tendon. This a very sensitive area and it may feel very tender to the dog. When you apply

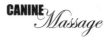

pressure to SP38, the dog might flinch and perhaps try to pull away from the pressure. If the point is very tender you might see some skin twitching along the hindquarters and he might flex the knee (stifle) on the same side. This is a sign of excessive tightness and stress; if you feel heat under your fingers, suspect inflammation. The whole muscle might show tightness along its course, proportional to the severity of the muscular stress. If the stress point is well defined, consider also working the tendon of insertion using the "origin-insertion" technique.

39. The Digital Extensor Muscles: *Extend Paw During Movement*

Located in the superficial layer, these muscles originate on the distal femur and proximal tibia. They run distally to insert on the anterior aspect of the tarsal bones and digits. Their contraction causes the tarsus to flex and the digits to extend (dorsi flex).

When these muscles are tight, they will limit the protraction of the foreleg during motion, the regular stride will be somewhat shortened on that side. The retraction power will also be reduced. The dog shows discomfort upon palpation.

SP 39 is felt as a tight knot below its attachment point on the tibia. It may feel very tender to the dog. When you apply pressure to SP 39, the dog might flinch and perhaps try to pull away from the pressure, flexing the leg on the same side. If the point is very tender you might see some skin twitching along the leg and shoulder muscles. This is a sign of excessive tightness and stress; if you feel heat under your fingers, suspect inflammation. The whole muscle group will feel tight along its course, proportional to the severity of the mus-

cular stress. If the stress point is well defined, consider also working the tendon of insertion using the "origin-insertion" technique.

40. The Digital Flexor Muscles: *Flex Paw During Movement*

Located in the superficial layer, these muscles originate on the distal femur and proximal tibia and fibula. They run distally to insert on the posterior aspect of the tarsal bones and digits. Their contraction causes the tarsus to extend and the digits to flex.

When these muscles are tight, they will limit the flexion of the foreleg during motion, the regular stride will be somewhat shortened on that side. The protraction motion will also be affected. The dog shows discomfort upon palpation.

SP 40 is felt as a tight knot by the origin attachment point next to the fibula on the medial aspect of the hind leg. It may feel very tender to the dog. When you apply pressure to SP 40, the dog might flinch and perhaps try to pull away from the pressure. If the point is very tender you might see some skin twitching along the leg muscles. This is a sign of excessive tightness and stress; if you feel heat under your fingers, suspect inflammation. The whole muscle will feel tight along its course, proportional to the severity of the muscular stress. If the stress point is well defined, consider also working the tendon of insertion using the "origin-insertion" technique.

Some activities that could cause stress on the hind quarters and hind legs are: ball chasing, squirrel chasing, agility competition, pulling a harness/cart/sled, hunting, tracking, guard dog training, herding, racing, Frisbee and flyball competition.

Remember that stress points usually develop in response to mechanical muscular stress during various activities, whether training, working or playing. When you find a stress point somewhere in the dog's musculature, most likely you will find some other stress points either close by as part of the same muscle groups involved in that particular movement, or in other adjacent muscle groups compensating for the actual discomfort. It is also important to keep in mind that a stress point can actually form in response to an external trauma or even a bad fall. Your palpation of the various afflicted structures will allow you to identify the knotted muscular areas as well as the compensatory muscle tension. For a better understanding of the compensatory factors in the dog's musculature please review the Chapter 3 on kinesiology of the dog.

Another important factor to keep in mind is that when a stress point forms, it often affects the local blood circulation to the muscles involved, causing the formation of trigger points as a result of lactic acid buildup in the contracted fibers. Be gentle in your massage application as you know the trigger points are very sensitive to the dog, as they are for us humans! For best performance in your massage work, you should from time to time thoroughly review the stress point massage technique and the trigger point massage technique discussed later.

Gait Assessment

You can train your eyes to detect muscular problems by closely watching the actions of your dog when walking, trotting or running. Assess the length of the strides, the smoothness of execution and the soundness of each step. If your dog

is lame in the front leg, it will raise or bob his head as the lame leg strikes the ground. If lame in the hind leg, your dog will drop his head as the lame leg strikes the ground. Any lameness during the walk shows a possible problem in the muscular structure. Generally, lameness during the trot indicates a structural problem and you should check with your veterinarian.

The Trouble Spots Massage Routine

The trouble spots routine is designed to deal with the most commonly occurring "trouble spot" areas of the dog, to prevent their corresponding stress points from developing as well as the eventual formation of trigger points. This routine is a nice complement to a maintenance routine especially if your animal exercises regularly.

If a strong level of inflammation is detected in these areas, first apply the ice cup massage technique for a few minutes to decrease the sensitivity of the nerve endings and reduce the inflammation. Begin your work with the short version of the relaxation routine to calm and prepare the dog. Follow with the trouble spot routine, starting at the neck with the first trouble spot area.

1. Work the entire upper neck area where the splenius and the upper rhomboideus muscles attach, as well as the ligamentum nuchae attachment at the occiput between the ears and behind the skull. This is an area of constant stress for a dog who engages in strenuous activities. Use the SEW approach to warm up the whole upper neck. Take the time to relax the muscles fibers in that area with lots of thumb kneadings and gentle finger frictions; this work will prevent the formation of SP 1 and SP 2. Then apply some muscle squeezing along the crest of the neck start-

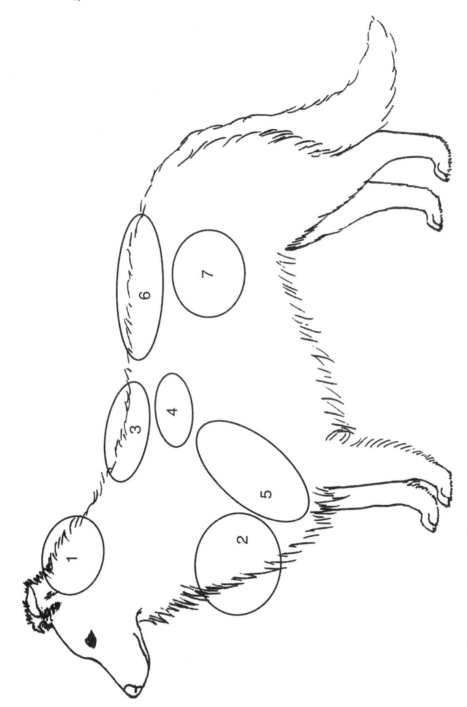

8.14 The Trouble Spots Massage Routine Outline

ing with a five pound pressure and progressing to 10 pounds depending on the degree of tension you find; use your judgment.

If the area is tender, the dog will react by moving away from the pressure or by arching the neck against your pressure. If you move too quickly into heavier pressure you may make the existing tension worse. Use the WES approach to drain the neck and flow to the next trouble spot.

2. In the lower aspect of the neck, the next trouble spot is found in the cleidocephalicus muscle. This muscle is involved in the protraction of the foreleg, the head carriage and side movements of the neck and head. If the cleidocephalicus muscle becomes tight, the dog will not be able to carry its head correctly and it will be uncomfortable when circling. Severe tightening of this muscle results in the dog being off on most of its movements.

When the muscle is tender, the animal will react to light pressure by flinching and pulling away. As you work this area, the dog will most likely relax into the treatment and drop his neck and shoulder on the same side you are treating.

To massage this area, start with the SEW approach over the neck from top to bottom. Then apply kneadings to loosen the muscle fibers and prevent the formation of SP 3. Follow with some gentle cross-fiber frictions over the whole length of the muscle. Intersperse with thorough effleurages to drain the area. Then apply gentle compressions to the entire length of the muscle. Follow with the WES approach to drain the neck thoroughly and finish with some light strokings flowing to the next trouble spot.

3. The withers area is the skeletal attachment site for the rhomboideus and the trapezius muscles which are directly involved in the movement of the scapula. The repetitive movement of any gait and the stress of a potentially difficult maneuver (for example, the impact of landing after a jump) in combination with poor footing can cause irritation of the muscle attachment onto the withers.

As you reach this area with strokings, move on to warm up the muscles with the SEW approach. Then use gentle muscle squeezing to assess the degree of inflammation or irritation. Thoroughly drain the area with lots of effleurages, use kneadings to loosen the muscle fibers then drain with effleurages again. Apply gentle friction across the length of the fibers starting gently with moderate pressure and rhythm, working progressively deeper for a period of two minutes. This will prevent the formation of SP 6, 7 and 8. Intersperse with effleurages every 20 seconds to drain the area as you work. Keep track of time to avoid overworking the fibers. Follow with the WES approach to ensure a generous drainage. Finish with light strokings and move over to check the fourth "trouble spot."

4. The anterior attachment of the longissimus dorsi is located behind the withers a few inches down from the top of the withers. Irritation and inflammation of this area can result from an extensive workout.

When this area is irritated, tension can be felt in one or both sides of this muscle and will eventually lead to the formation of SP 5 and SP 20. Take time to warm up the area with the SEW approach over the whole muscle. Then use kneadings to relax the muscle fibers and follow with some gentle finger frictions to prevent the formation of SP5. If sore, the dog will probably flinch, arch his back or move away from your pressure — the degree of reaction is indicative of the amount of inflammation present. If you detect a strong level of inflammation, apply the ice massage technique for a few minutes to decrease the sensitivity of the nerve endings while reducing the inflammation. Follow with light finger frictions along the entire muscle to loosen its fibers and intersperse with effleurages every 20 seconds. When finished, use the WES approach to thoroughly drain the whole muscle and then use light strokings to move to the next "trouble spot."

5. The supraspinatus muscle is one of the most important muscles of the shoulder; it works in conjunction with the infraspinatus, the deltoideus and the teres major. These muscles serve to prevent lateral dislocation of the shoulder. The supraspinatus is directly involved in lateral movements such as abduction (as the agonist muscle) and adduction (as the antagonist muscle) of the foreleg. Abrupt changes of direction to the sides as might occur in herding or agility renders the supraspinatus very susceptible to strain. When the muscle is sore, the dog will exhibit signs of lameness and restricted movement in the foreleg on the same side.

Start massaging this area with the SEW approach. The dog may flinch or, if feeling very tender, will move away from your pressure. So start working lightly with lots of effleurages and wringings to warm up the area. Then apply light kneadings to relax the muscle fibers and follow with effleurages. Friction the entire muscle, back and forth for two minutes to loosen its fibers; this will prevent the formation of SP 9 and SP 10. Intersperse with effleurages every 20 seconds. Follow with gentle compressions to the entire length of the muscle and finish with the WES approach to thoroughly drain the entire muscle. Use strokings to move to the next "trouble spot."

6. The longissimus dorsi (caudal attachment) and the middle gluteal muscle join in this area which is most often found to be very sensitive. Start massaging the area delicately with the SEW approach. When the area is inflamed or knotted, the dog will sink or sag in response to your pressure. Apply the ice massage technique first to numb the nerve endings of the area you are treating. Then stimulate the circulation thoroughly with wringings and gentle compressions. Intersperse with effleurages every 20 seconds. Use kneadings to relax the muscles fibers. Follow with light frictions along the entire muscles to prevent the formation of SP 20 and SP 21. Thoroughly drain the area with effleurages. Apply palmar compressions along the length of the whole muscles to complete the treatment. Finish with the WES approach to thoroughly drain the area. Use light strokings to move to the next trouble spot.

7. The hip attachment of the tensor fasciae latae (TFL) area just below the point of the hip is a very critical spot. This is where both the TFL muscle and the iliopsoas muscle originate. These two muscles are strong hip flexors. Furthermore the TFL muscle plays a role in extending the stifle during retraction of the hind leg.

When this trouble-spot area is stressed, the dog will show discomfort on the same side when turning and will tend to throw his leg outward during protraction. Be careful and very gentle when starting to work this area. If the area appears very tender at first touch, use the ice massage technique prior to the treatment to numb the nerve endings. Stir up the circulation in the area with the SEW approach. Apply compressions with a moderate to heavy pressure (5 to 12 pounds) along the TFL muscle. Then use kneadings to relax the muscle fibers and prevent the formation of SP 36 and SP

37, intersperse with effleurages. Apply cross-fiber frictions over the entire muscle to loosen the muscle fibers. Alternate with some effleurages every 20 seconds. After the massage, apply cold to ease the nerve endings and flush the blood circulation in that area. Finish with the WES approach to thoroughly drain the area.

To finish this routine, apply lots of light stroking over the entire dog's body to give it a sense of relaxation. Complete you massage with a general stretching routine of the dog which is particularly good to contribute to the positive effect of your massage work. After this massage routine, some light exercising for the dog is recommended as a good follow-up, but keep any lateral work (circles) to a minimum at first, especially if the shoulder and TFL muscles were tight.

Stretching

CHAPTER 9

This chapter will explain the benefits of stretching and demonstrate the stretching exercises that you can add to your massage practice. Dogs stretch spontaneously and naturally, tuning up their muscles and keeping their joints flexible. In normal conditions, a dog will not overstretch. Regular stretching can prevent muscle problems, provide relaxation and develop your dog's body awareness. Stretching will improve your dog's coordination as well as give you feedback on his physical condition. It is important to note that if your dog has had any recent physical problems such as a fall, direct trauma or surgery, particularly of the joints and muscles, If so, please consult your veterinarian before you start a stretching program.

The benefits of regular stretching exercises are both physical and cerebral.

Physical Benefits

The apparent musculoskeletal benefit of frequent stretching exercises result in increased flexibility, in prevention of injuries, in improved general metabolism and in better movement.

- **Flexibility**: Stretching keeps the muscle fibers and the joints flexible. When you stretch a muscle, you lengthen its fibers. This action mechanically affects the "Golgi sensory" nerve cells and the "muscle spindle" sensory nerve cells, resetting the feedback mechanism to the central nervous system. The results are vasodilation and tonification of the fibers. Stretching also improves the tone of the muscle fibers and the elasticity of the ligaments and the joint capsules. Stretching reduces muscle tension and therefore prevents muscle pulls. A strong, pre-stretched muscle resists stress better than a strong, unstretched muscle. Better elasticity of the muscles, tendons and ligaments allows for freer, easier, more controlled and quicker movements—all resulting in better overall coordination.

- **Prevention of injuries**: Stretching not only prevents muscle strain, ligament sprain and loosens the joint capsules, but also makes the body feel more relaxed.

It releases muscle contracture due to old scar tissue, helps relieve muscle pain from chronic tension and reduces post-exercise soreness and stiffness.

- **Metabolism**: Muscle stretching increases blood and lymph circulation and brings more oxygen and nutrients to the body parts. It also prevents inflammation and scar tissue formation, trigger point formation, and stress point build-up.

- **Improvements**: Regular stretching will improve the range of motion of the joints, the stride's length, the overall coordination and the response time of the reflexes. The physiological benefits of stretching exercises upon the body are immediate. You should regularly add them to your massage work.

Cerebral Benefits

A dog's "body awareness" is, of course, cerebral or mental. Hence, one part of stretching is cerebral because the activity develops body awareness via the nervous system. As you stretch various body parts, you help your dog to focus on them and to become mentally in touch with them. This process develops the animal's self-awareness thereby improving coordination in all aspects of movement.

The stretching of muscles sends relaxation impulses—via sensory nerves—to the central nervous system, reflexively loosening the dog's mind control over his body. Stretching will also decrease motor nerve tension transmitted throughout the body. The animal will relax both physically and mentally, an important message

factor when dealing with animals who have been in accidents, have been frightened or are in pain. Stretching will indirectly help dogs to release the anxiety associated with muscle tension.

Stretching will give you feedback on the state of health of the muscle groups and of the ligament structures, particularly in regards to their elasticity and tone.

When to Stretch

Warning! Always stretch when the dog is warm.

Muscles, tendons and ligaments and eventually joint capsules risk damage if stretched when cold. Stretching a dog after a warm up (walk/trot) period will limit the risk of injury from overstretching. It is best to stretch as cool-downs immediately after playing or training. Again, if your animal has had any recent physical problems or surgery, particularly of the joints and muscles, or if he has been inactive or sedentary for some time, consult your veterinarian before you start a stretching program.

Observing the warning just given, you can stretch your dog at any time. Stretching should be done every day, after every playing or training session, and should be included with your massage work. A regular routine will give you feedback on the physical condition of your dog, the flexibility of his joints, the agility of his muscle groups, the progression of the animal's training program and the effects of your massage treatments.

If you need to stretch a specific area during a localized massage treatment for a handicapped dog, that area can be warmed up with a hot towel, a hot hard pack or simply by massage.

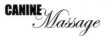

The Stretch Reflex

The stretch reflex is a protective mechanism which prevents a muscle from being overstretched and torn. The stretch reflex is a nervous reaction caused when the muscle spindle, a sensory nerve cell, is overstretched. When overstretched, the muscle spindle fires nerve impulses to the spinal cord. The reflex arc mechanism located in the spine then fires back motor nerve impulses that cause an instant muscle contraction. This contraction prevents the muscle from being injured. So, do not overstretch, do not try to reach beyond the muscle's maximum flexibility. Instead, just hold the stretch in a relaxed manner and for a longer period of time. The dog's flexibility will increase naturally when you start stretching regularly.

How to Stretch

To attain best results, you need to respect the structures you are working on. To manipulate correctly, it is important to be concerned with the animal's natural body alignment. Always move and stretch the dog's limb in their natural range of motion. Do not exert torque or an abnormal twist.

Stretching is not a contest to see how far you can stretch, or how much more you can stretch each time. The object of stretching is to relax muscle and ligament tension in order to promote freer movement and to trigger the other benefits listed earlier. To achieve all of this, you need to stretch safely, starting with the easy stretch described in this chapter and building to a regular, deeper stretch. Never go too far, the stretch reflex will cause the muscle to contract to prevent tearing of the fibers.

Stretching should always be done in a relaxed and steady manner. The first time you stretch your dog, do it slowly and gently. Give the dog time to adjust its body and mind to the physical and the nervous stress release that stretching initiates. The stretch should be tailored to the animal's particular muscular structure, flexibility and varying tension levels. Again, because you will risk tearing the muscle and ligament fibers, do not overstretch.

When you release a stretch, gently return the leg in its original position. Note that many dogs show varying degrees of sensitivity to handling. Understand that how you handle your dog from the beginning has a very definite impact on how you will be able to handle it in the future. Make a distinction between a reaction to pain and an objection to handling.

The Easy Stretch

Always start with the easy stretch. The easy stretch means stretching only 75 to 80 percent of the total stretching capability of that particular body part and holding it only for 10 to 20 seconds. Your dog will enjoy this gentle approach. Be steady in the development of your work. Never work hastily or with jerky movements. Do not pull excessively on the leg because you risk tearing muscle fibers by overstretching.

For example, take hold of your dog's foreleg gently and guide it through its forward range of motion, bringing it to its natural point of stretch. There you should feel a mild tension and at that point release your traction slightly. That is the easy stretch. Be relaxed as you hold the stretch.

Hold the position for 10 seconds during which the tension should subside. Then gently return the leg to its natural position.

The Deeper Stretch

Once the dog gets used to the easy stretch, you can work into the deeper stretch. Start with the easy stretch. After the initial 10 seconds, and as the muscle tightness decreases, adjust your traction until you again feel a mild tension. Hold for another five seconds. If your dog does not mind, repeat two to three times until you feel you have reached the maximum stretching capacity of the muscle. Do not exceed one minute on any given stretch. Avoid triggering the stretch reflex by overstretching. Be in control.

Spontaneous Stretch

Often during the development stretch and sometimes during the easy stretch, the dog will spontaneously stretch himself fully for a few seconds. This is a definite sign that the animal is enjoying the stretch and that it needs it very much. As you hold the limb during such spontaneous release, you can feel all the deep tension coming out as a vibration; it is quite an experience. After such a release, there is no need to hold the stretch further. Bring the limb back to its natural position.

Mental Counting

The time frame in which you stretch a muscle is very important. At first, silently count the seconds for each stretch. This will ensure that you hold tension for the correct length of time. After a while, you will develop a feel for this practice and will subconsciously know when the animal has reached its full stretching capability without having to count. This practice of mental counting will help you get the best results from the stretching technique. Be aware of the dog's reaction to the stretch before you repeat the exercise. You should also investigate if any undue stress points or trigger points are present; release them with the proper massage technique.

General Stretching Outline

First start with the easy stretch for 10 to 15 seconds, then work into the deeper stretch. This activity will finely tune the muscles and increase overall flexibility. Do not overstretch, do not make jerky or bouncy movements. Never stretch an acutely or recently torn muscle. Never force the joint in any abnormal range or twist it. Always stretch the agonist muscle and its antagonist muscle. A regular practice of stretching with comfortable and painless movements will help you go beyond your animal's current flexibility limit and come closer to its full potential.

The Stretching Routine

The Foreleg Stretches

There are three foreleg stretches: the forward stretch, the backward stretch, and shoulder rotation.

The Forward Stretch

This protraction movement will stretch the muscles involved in the retraction of the foreleg. Pick up the leg above the paw with one hand and place the other behind the elbow. Gently bring the leg forward and upward. This stretch will affect the muscles of the shoulder, the trapezius, the rhomboideus, the latissimus dorsi, the serratus cervicis, the deltoid and the triceps. Once the dog is well into the stretch, maintain the tension with one hand behind and above the wrist, and with your other hand extend the paw. This action will deepen the stretch of the flexor tendons. Be gentle and cautious.

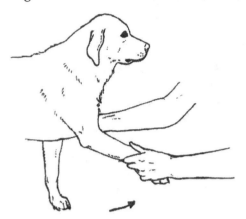

9.1   Foreleg Forward Stretch

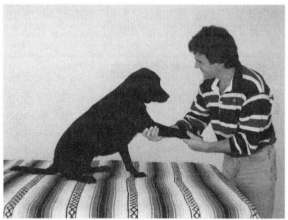

9.2   Foreleg Forward Stretch

The Backward Stretch

The retraction movement will stretch the muscles involved in the protraction of the foreleg. With one hand, pick up the leg above the paw. Place the other hand in front and below the elbow joint.

Gently bring the leg backward until the radius bone is slightly past the 90 degree angle with the ground. This is a good stretch for the muscle of the chest and the upper leg, specifically, the pectorals, the brachiocephalicus, the biceps and the extensors.

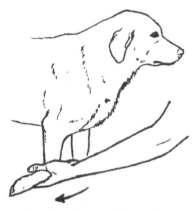

9.3   Foreleg Backward Stretch

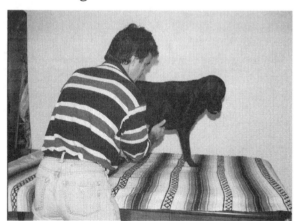

9.4   Foreleg Backward Stretch

Once the dog is well into the stretch, maintain the tension with one hand in front and above the wrist, and with your other hand flex the paw. This action will deepen the stretch of the extensor tendons. Be gentle and cautious.

The Shoulder Rotation

The following variation will help loosen deep muscles such as the pectorals, the serratus cervicis and thoracis, the intercostal fascia and to relax the ligaments and muscles of the shoulder girdle structure. Slide one hand between the chest and the forearm, and with your other hand grab gently the lower foreleg above the paw. Start a circular movement moving the leg inward, then forward, outward and back. Repeat three to five times then reverse the movement. Avoid excessive pressure at the shoulder joint.

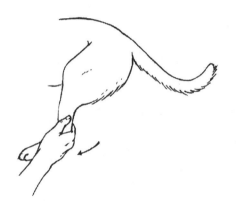

9.5 Hind Leg Forward Stretch

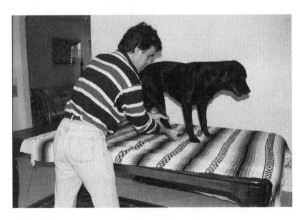

9.6 Hind Leg Forward Stretch

The Hind Leg Stretches

There are three hind leg stretches: the forward stretch, the backward stretch, and the hind leg transverse stretch.

The Forward Stretch

This protraction movement—also known as the hamstring stretch—will stretch the muscles involved in the retraction of the hind leg. With one hand, pick up the paw. Position your other hand below and behind the hock joint, and gently move the leg forward in its natural line of movement. While the leg is forward you may consider moving it a little inward. Do not move the hind leg to the outside because this is not a natural movement; it could adversely affect the hip joint. This is a good stretch for the muscles of the hip and thighs, the tensor fascia latae, the gluteus and the hamstring muscles (the semi-tendinosus, the semi-membranosus and the biceps femoris). Once comfortable in the stretch, you can consider extending the paw to deepen the stretch over the flexor tendons. Be gentle and cautious.

The Backward Stretch

This retraction movement will stretch the muscles involved in the flexion of the hip and of the leg. With one hand pick up the paw and place

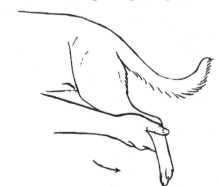

9.7 Hind Leg Backward Stretch

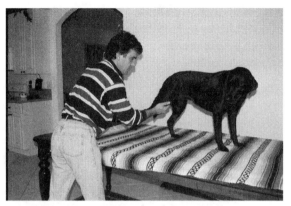

9.8 Hind Leg Backward Stretch

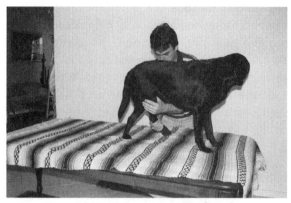

9.10 Hind Leg Transverse Stretch

your other hand in front of the hock joint. Bring the leg back through its natural range until you feel the stretch. Once comfortable in the stretch, you can consider flexing the paw to deepen the stretch over the extensor tendons. Be gentle and cautious. This is a good stretch for the following muscles: the iliacus, the sartorius, the tensor fascia latae, the quadriceps femoris, the extensor and the abdominal muscles.

The Hind Leg Transverse Stretch

This is another movement to stretch the quadriceps femoris muscle of the hind leg and the TFL muscle. Grasp the rear leg above the paw on the

opposite side of the dog and bring the leg under the belly and slightly toward opposite front paw. Be aware of the torque you will produce on the hock and the stifle joint by stretching this way. Do not apply too much pressure. Be gentle, paying attention to your dog's comfort.

The Back Muscles

There is no particular stretching movement for the back muscles. But by reflex, you can affect these muscles if you press your thumb into the belly region, right over the attachment tendon of the pectoralis minor profondus muscle on

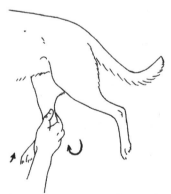

9.9 Hind Leg Transverse Stretch

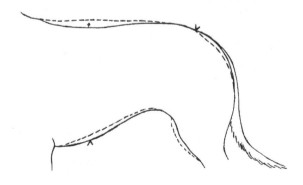

9.11 Back Muscle Stretch

the sternum bone. This will cause the dog to tuck up, thereby rounding its back and stretching these muscles: longissimus dorsi, iliocostalis and the spinalis dorsi. Also tickling the belly will cause the same reflex. This is one of the easiest stretches.

Another way to affect these muscles is to stimulate the sacrum area along its edges with some thumb point pressure moves. This will cause a reflex action in the abdominal muscles which will result in an arching of the back structure and a stretching of the back muscles.

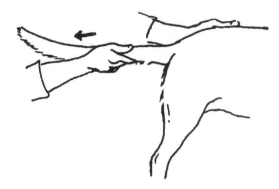

9.13   Tail Stretch

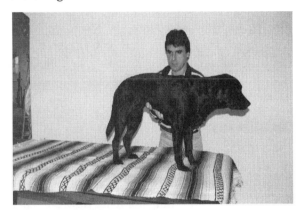

9.12   Back Muscle Stretch

The Tail Stretch

Stretching the tail is a great way to produce a feeling of deep relaxation in your dog. This stretch is a major part of the relaxation massage routine. When approaching the rear, use gentle strokings along the tail bone and down the buttocks before picking up the tail with one of your hands. Leave your other hand on the sacrum. Take hold of the tail a few inches from its base and gently move it in a circle starting clockwise, two or three times. Repeat in the anti-clockwise direction two

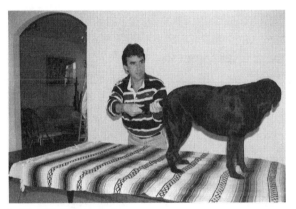

9.14   Tail Stretch

or three times. During these movements, take note of any restriction found in moving the tail to either side.

At this point, move to the back of the dog and very gently pull on the tail (1 to 2 pounds maximum, use common sense, don't pull to the point of discomfort). Hold this stretch for approximately one minute unless the dog shows discomfort. Usually the dog, feeling good, responds positively by pulling against your traction or lowering its head.

Using light muscle squeezing moves between the thumb and fingers of your right hand, gently squeeze each vertebra from the base of the tail down. Keep stretching with the left hand. Reverse hands if that is more suitable to you. Make note of the tail's flexibility looking for sore spots and possible inflammation. Release the stretch progressively and then stroke the hind quarters and sacrum area for a few seconds.

If the dog shows discomfort, inflammation or abnormal symptoms with palpation of this area prior to your stretching, the stretching would be contraindicated. Check with your veterinarian.

Neck Stretches

These neck stretches will affect all aspects of the neck's muscles. You can do all stretches using an incentive such as a piece of dog biscuit. This makes the work much, much easier.

Lateral Stretch

Allow the dog to sniff the "incentive" and guide it towards the side/back. This movement will stretch the neck's extensor and flexor muscles

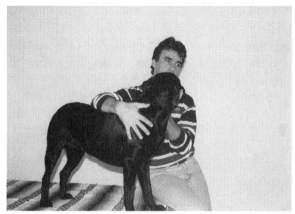

9.16 Lateral Neck Stretch

on the opposite side. You can increase the lateral stretch by asking your dog to stretch further towards the point of the hip. Talk softly to your animal as you get it into the stretch. Do both the right and left sides.

Neck Flexion Stretch

As with the lateral stretch, use an incentive to guide your dog's head down in between its legs. In performing this particular stretch, you can add a variation: as you bring the head down move its head either to the right or to the left. The exten-

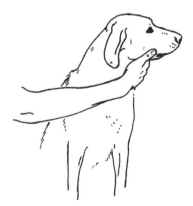

9.15 Lateral Neck Stretch

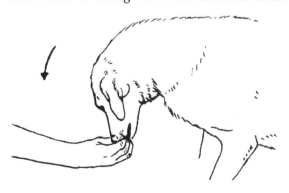

9.17 Neck Flexion Stretch

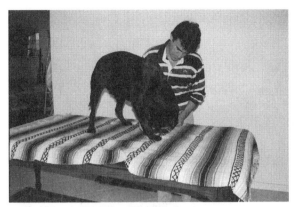

9.18 Neck Flexion Stretch

sor muscles will thus be thoroughly stretched. For maximum benefits, insure your dog does not flex his elbows during this stretch.

Neck Extension Stretch

As with the other neck stretches, use an incentive to guide your dog's head upward and out as far as it can go. This movement will stretch the neck's flexor muscles.

Regular stretching exercises will contribute greatly to the dog's overall flexibility and fitness. They should be part of its regular exercise program. Done individually, stretching will assist you in the application and success of your massage treatments.

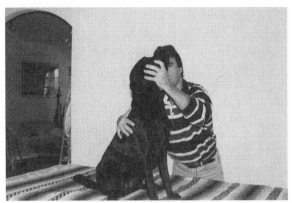

9.20 Neck Extension Stretch

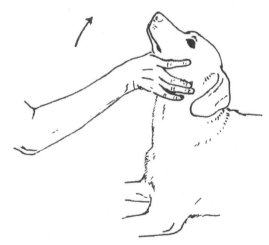

9.19 Neck Extension Stretch

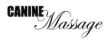

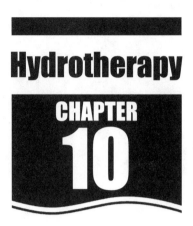

Hydrotherapy

CHAPTER 10

This section explains the benefits and demonstrates the application of hydrotherapy, which means water treatment applied externally to the body. The name hydrotherapy is taken from the Greek words *hydros* meaning water and *therapia* meaning treatment. Using hydrotherapy before and after massage treatments will increase the effectiveness of your work.

Heat and cold are used to relieve pain in acute or chronic conditions and in inflammatory disorders for both humans and animals. Heat and cold are still the best treatment in the practice of pain control. No other methods are as effective, as safe and easy to use, as free from side effects and as cost effective. Because they affect the cutaneous nerve endings, both heat and cold decrease pain and muscle tension. Accomplished through opposite physical effects, they are used at different stages of an injury's development such as cold in the acute stage, and heat for chronic conditions.

Hydrotherapy comes in a number of forms depending upon the temperature of the water, the method of application, the duration of treatment and so on. Whenever you apply hydrotherapy to your dog, always monitor the entire process, checking feedback signs at all times, being ready to adjust your treatment if any discomfort arises.

Water applications produce two effects: a first, temporary effect and a second, more lasting effect. For example, cold first constricts the blood vessels and numbs the nerve endings for pain control. Then, it triggers a lasting dilation of the vessels. Heat first dilates the blood vessels and soothes the nerve endings; then, it causes a lasting relaxation of the tissues.

Water application temperatures are classified as:

Cold	40 to 60°F (4.4 to 15.5°C)
Cool	65 to 75°F (18.3 to 23.8°C)
Tepid	85 to 95°F (29.4 to 35°C)
Warm	90 to 100°F (32.2 to 37.7°C)
Hot	100 to 110°F (37.7 to 43.3°C)

WARNING! For hot applications, the temperature should be 5 to 12°C (41 to 53.6°F) above normal body temperature which is about 38°C (100.4°F).

Water temperatures between 43 and 50°C (109.4 to 122°F) should be safe. Above 50°C, 122°F, you risk burning the skin. Use a thermometer to be sure; it is better to be safe than sorry.

Duration of Treatment

The more extreme the temperature, the shorter the application's duration; the more moderate the temperature, the more prolonged the application. A very short duration is about five to 15 seconds, a short duration is between 15 and 60 seconds, an average duration is about two minutes, a prolonged duration is between three and 10 minutes, a very prolonged duration is from 10 to 30 minutes.

Stages of Recovery

In therapy, there are three stages in the recovery process of an injury: the acute stage, the sub-acute stage and the chronic stage. These definitions are not precise as there are also in-between stages.

The Acute Stage

The first 24 hours following an injury is the acute stage. Use cold immediately. This will stop hemorrhaging in the damaged tissues and will contribute to reducing the swelling before you commence massage. You can apply cold as ice in a solid form or crushed with some water in a plastic bag or as cold running water.

The Sub-Acute Stage

The time between 24 and 72 hours is considered the sub-acute stage. By then, depending on the severity, the injury has usually stabilized. Use the vascular flush—alternating cold and heat applications—several minutes for each application. Immediately after a massage, you may apply some cold to sooth tender tissues.

The In-Between Stages

Closer to the acute stage, in the first 24 to 48 hours, first apply cold for three minutes, then apply heat for two minutes. Repeat this cycle two to three times. Always finish with cold. Follow with a light effleurage toward the heart or simply use stroking if the body part appears to be too sensitive.

When closer to the chronic stage—48 to 72 hours —first apply heat for three minutes, then apply cold for two minutes. Repeat two to three times. **Always finish with cold for two minutes.** Follow with a light effleurage toward the heart or use light stroking if the body part appears to be too sensitive.

The Chronic Stage

Beyond 72 hours, in the chronic stage, use heat to loosen the tissues and to increase blood circulation. After a massage, you may apply some cold to soothe the tender tissues, especially if you have worked them deeply.

When an old chronic injury flares up, soreness with some degree of inflammation and eventually some swelling may occur at the site. In this case, use cold hydrotherapy to relieve the edema and numb the irritated nerve endings. This action will reduce the inflammation and allow you to work more easily. You may use a vascular flush as well, always finishing with cold.

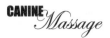

Consider the situation carefully. If you choose to use cold water over a large area, as in a case of inflammation of the back, do not apply it if the dog is cold or chilled. Help your dog warm up first with a short walk or play. However, if a cold water treatment is to be used over a local area as in a case of tendonitis, the warming up of that area can simply be achieved by massage (wringings and effleurages).

Cold

Cold is widely used in emergencies - right after an injury or a trauma — to stop any bleeding, prevent excessive swelling and lower the pain level. Cold can also be applied during the flare-up of old chronic injuries to reduce inflammation and pain symptoms.

Effects of Cold

Cold water application first chills the skin. This causes the constriction of the blood capillaries, the lymph channels, the muscular and the elastic tissues contained in the dermis. This constriction drives the blood to the interior, reducing circulation and preventing swelling in the trauma area. Cold also decreases pain by numbing the sensory nerve endings.

After the cold is removed, there comes a secondary reaction. The blood capillaries expand, allowing blood to return to the body's surface. This reaction is the body's defense mechanism responding to warm the entire body. If the treatment is applied to the entire body, circulation will be stimulated over the entire system. This stimulation will raise the body's temperature, increase skin activity, raise the blood pressure, contract the muscles, strengthen the heart action, stimulate the nervous system, stimulate the metabolism and will slow and deepen breathing.

Prolonged cool applications produces similar effects to cold, but these are not as marked and the reaction is thus not quite as pronounced.

Application of Cold

Ice packs and other cold applications may be used for contusions and sprains during the first 24 hours. Cold reduces hemorrhaging and swelling in the damaged fibers. It also contributes to controlling pain by activating endorphin production.

In treating acute problems be careful not to lower the temperature too much by excessive cold or prolonged water treatments. A "cold reaction" may follow. Cover the dog with a blanket.

Cold is also used in chronic cases to decrease pain in very tender areas or to reduce the swelling in a chronically inflamed area (for example, tendonitis, bursitis, arthritis). By absorbing heat from the irritated area, cold reduces the metabolic rate thereby keeping the inflammation low, reducing the incidence of muscle spasm and reducing nerve irritation by slowing down the velocity of nerve conduction. All of this breaks the pain-spasm-pain cycle. Cold is used extensively in the control of inflamed tendons and joint structures.

Cold water should be used to relieve burn pain. Immediately immerse the burned area in very cold or ice water, or spray cold water over the area until the animal is pain free. Check with your veterinarian.

Cold Devices and Techniques

Several cooling devices are used in cold therapy:

- Specially designed leg wraps with Velcro containing chemical ice bags. These leg wraps are easy to assemble and are very convenient when traveling.

- Specially designed leg boots that can be filled with cold water.

- The most widely known and very practical application is "frozen slush." To prepare it, mix one part of Isoprophyl alcohol in three parts of water in a zip-lock bag and leave in the freezer. When ready, apply as needed. It is re-usable indeed.

- Containers of cold water are very practical and popular. To remove toxins from the skin and keep swelling down some practitioners add apple cider vinegar and sea salt.

- Crushed ice and water in a plastic bag wrapped in a towel, applied to the skin and held with a bandage is very practical, easy to prepare and inexpensive.

- Cold poultices are very effective in relieving tendon inflammation. They are made with a semi-solid mixture of clay in a cotton cloth and applied to the body part cold.

- A cotton towel wrung out in cold water and kept in a refrigerator or freezer can be wrapped around a leg or joint to reduce inflammation. Hold in place with a leg wrap or pin.

- A cold towel or a cold mitten applied with large friction movements over the whole body will produce a stimulating, tonic effect.

- Sponging with cool water is a quick way to cool off a dog during exercise.

- Pools are great for water exercises.

The Ice Cup Massage Technique

Use a four to eight ounce paper or Styrofoam cup, filled with water and frozen. Hold the cup by the bottom, peel the rim away and apply the ice on the coat to massage the area in a circular motion. The rhythm should not be too slow, nor too fast, approximately four seconds for every five inch circle. The pressure is light, one or two pounds. The application should last for one to two minutes for small dogs and up to five minutes maximum for a large dog. Observe the structure, the degree of swelling, the inflammation present in the tissues and the tenderness of the tissues. Be careful not to cause ice burns. Follow with a light massage (strokings, effleurages, gentle kneadings)

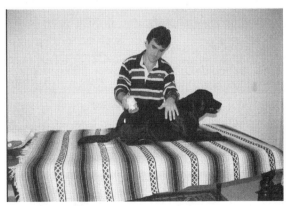

10.1 Ice Cup Massage Technique

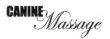

or wrap the area with some cloth to regenerate warmth quickly. This technique is very useful when dealing with any swelling and inflammation in the leg. It is easily available, easily transported, easily applicable and is inexpensive.

Duration of Cold Application

Cold should be applied for a prolonged duration, lasting approximately 10 minutes, but no longer than 12 minutes. Direct ice application such as ice massage should be of average duration. It should not last more than two or three minutes when applied directly over a thin coat, or up to five minutes when over a thick coat. When using cold on an open bleeding wound, do not apply it for more than 10 minutes because it will interfere with the blood's coagulation process. Use a short duration, two or three minutes application, for very sensitive body parts such as the face or groin.

Cold hydrotherapy applications are easily available, easy to work with, inexpensive and very effective. Have some ice cups and wet towels ready for use in your freezer. It pays to be ready for emergencies! Include this procedure in your preventive therapy, before and after your massages; it will make your work easier and more effective.

Heat

Heat is invaluable in therapy. Heat is used at every level in the medical practice - not only in hydrotherapy, but also with ultrasound, lasers, heating lamps and so on. In combination with massage therapy, heat greatly helps in the recovery stages of injuries, as well as in maintenance and preventive programs.

Effects of Heat

Heat first decreases pain by soothing the sensory nerve endings. Heat causes vasodilation of blood and lymph channels resulting in improved circulation, bringing more oxygen and nutrients to the structures, as well as assisting in the removal of toxins. Heat loosens fibers (muscle, tendon, ligament), dislodges toxins and prepares the subject area for a good massage. Moist heat is more effective than dry heat because it penetrates more deeply into the body.

Another effect of heat is to bring a general feeling of relaxation to the muscle fibers, tendons and ligaments. Heat raises the body temperature, increases skin activity, stimulates the metabolism and lowers the blood pressure.

Application of Heat

Heat is used mostly in sub-acute or chronic cases of post traumatic recovery. Heat is used to soften the aches of old wounds, to ease low-grade inflammations, and to relieve stiffness in older animals. Used widely in deep massage treatments, heat loosens muscle fibers and other fibrous tissues prior to friction moves.

Heat may be used to control pain in acute injuries. If heat is used on contusions, sprains and other acute injuries, it should be as hot as can be tolerated, usually above 48°C (118°F). At higher temperatures, heat works as effectively as ice packs because of its great ability to stop bleeding into the tissues.

Heat Devices and Techniques

• A hot water bottle is very effective and practical to access.

• Heat lamps are efficient but require special installations.

• Electrical heating pads are not recommended. They may cause burns on recumbent patients and are potentially dangerous because they are a chewing hazard and a water shock (urine) hazard.

• Hydrocollator packs are probably the most convenient. These packs contain mud and are preheated in hot water containers. Wrap them in a towel before you apply them to your dog. Be careful that the temperature is not so high that it burns the animal's skin - no more than 12°C/53.6°F above normal body temperature.

• Hot towels are very convenient but need to be replaced regularly. Penetrating deeper into the muscle layers, wet or moist heat is generally more effective than dry heat. When applying hot towels, cover them with plastic to ensure an accumulation of body heat.

• Poultices are very effective. Poultices produce moist heat from a semi-solid mixture of various substances such as clay, flax seed or mustard applied to the body while hot.

• A hot water hosing application is very practical and popular.

• Some facilities are equipped with warm whirlpools. These are excellent for therapeutic exercises and training but are not easy to access.

• Counter-irritant liniments produce heat effectively, but they should be used very cautiously. Ask you veterinarian first, because there is a risk of skin irritation. Also, such liniment applications should be covered to prevent the dog from licking the product off or rubbing it into its eyes, etc.

Duration of Heat Application

Prolonged to very prolonged applications of 10 to 20 minutes are the rule for temperatures under 48°C/110°F. Because of the risk of overheating, no more than 20 minutes should be applied at a time. Heat above 48°C/110°F should be applied very carefully and for only a very short duration of from five to 15 seconds.

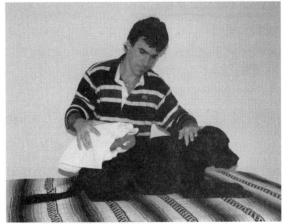

10.2 Heat Application -
Hot water bottle application.

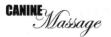

Too much heat applied too long can irritate nerve endings and result in neuralgia, a dull to severe ache in the nerve endings. If you suspect such a case has arisen, use cool cloths to numb those nerve endings and to bring back normal sensations. Also remember that a dog with a thick coat of hair may be a little insensitive to heat applied externally.

Heat is not as accessible as cold, but it is a great addition to your massage practice. Very useful in recovery treatment and in maintenance programs, heat is an easy and inexpensive way to tremendously improve your effectiveness. Acquire the necessary equipment and use it.

The use of water applications will greatly enhance your work and bring a lot of comfort to your animal. When well organized, they are a quick and inexpensive form of therapy to add to your massage routines.

Inflammation, Scar Tissue, Injuries & Common Problems

CHAPTER 11

Massage can greatly assist your dog during recovery from various injuries or common musculoskeletal problems. Always consult your veterinarian first for proper diagnosis in any situation and check the list of contraindications in Chapter 1 before applying any form of massage.

It is very important for you to understand the natural process of inflammation present in tissues following an injury. This will help you recognize the typical symptoms and to develop a better "finesse" of touch, improving your palpation skills. It is also important to know how to assess a scar as it is the end result of most inflammatory processes in the body.

Inflammation

Inflammation is the body's natural response to irritation such as bacteria, chemicals or heat, injury, virus or any other noxious phenomenon. It serves to destroy, dilute, or wall off both the injurious agent and the injured tissues so that repair may be effective. Inflammation's classical signs are: pain, heat, redness, swelling and loss of function and mobility.

There are three basic stages of inflammation:

First: The inflammatory process begins with a short period of vasoconstriction, followed quickly by a vasodilation with an increase in vascular permeability (swelling).

Second: Vasodilation allows fluids containing enzymes and other proteins to escape. This is followed by extravasion of PMN's (Polly Morphs Nucleotydes, aka Neutrophiles) and monocytes, which become macrophages. The enzymes and macrophages help to clear the wound of any debris.

Third: Repair begins with the deposit of fibrin in the vessels, the migration of fibroblasts to the area, and the eventual development of a scar. This process evolves over several hours to days depending on the severity of the inflammatory problem.

Within minutes after an injury, the dilation of the arterioles and the increased permeability produce heat, edema and redness (unfortunately not seen through the coat). As the local temperature rises slightly, the various metabolic reactions proceed

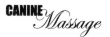

more rapidly and release additional heat. Excess edema results from increased permeability of blood vessels, which permits more fluid to move from blood to tissue spaces. Pain, whether immediate or delayed, is a cardinal symptom of inflammation and is responsible for limited movement if not complete immobility. Pain can result from the injury of nerve fibers, from irritation by toxic chemicals from micro-organisms, or from the increased pressure from excessive edema.

Although healing is initiated by local inflammation, excessive or prolonged inflammation may delay the healing and increase the scar formation potential. The severity, timing, and local character of any particular inflammatory response depend on its cause, the area affected, and the condition of the dog which in turn is influenced by nutrition, exercise levels, and age.

A chronic inflammatory process is a prolonged and persistent low-grade inflammation marked chiefly by new connective tissue formation, and occasional flare-ups with increased swelling.

Inflammatory problems can trigger associated degradation symptoms such as a general tenderness in the adjacent tissues (muscle groups, joint structure), compensatory muscle tension, and mood swings due to overall aching feeling when moving. Sometimes it is accompanied by loss of function.

Cold hydrotherapy is very beneficial for acute stages of inflammation during the first 12 to 24 hours, especially the ice-cup massage technique. Vascular flush is good for sub-acute stages. Heat is very efficient for chronic cases. Some chronic inflammations, especially if flaring up, benefit also from the use of cold applications.

Massage therapy is very beneficial to inflammation. Not always possible in the acute stage depending on the severity of symptoms, the swelling massage technique is very efficient in the sub-acute and chronic stages of inflammations. In the chronic stage, the myofascial technique is good to loosen the contracted fascia, and the friction technique is efficient to relieve the extra scar tissue formation.

Some Common Definitions Relating to Inflammation:

Myositis refers to the inflammation of a voluntary muscle.

Myositis fibrosa is an inflammation in which connective tissue forms within the muscle.

Myositis ossificans is a myositis marked by bony deposits or ossification of muscle.

Tendinitis refers to the inflammation of a tendon and of a tendon-muscle attachment.

Capsulitis refers to the inflammation of a joint capsule.

Synovitis refers to the inflammation of synovial membrane in a joint.

Tendinous synovitis refers to the inflammation of a tendon sheath.

Periostitis refers to the inflammation to the periosteum, covering of the bone.

Bursitis refers to the inflammation of a bursa.

Calcific bursitis refers to the inflammation and calcification of a bursa (very painful).

Fasciitis refers to the inflammation of the fascia.

Cases of inflammation caused by infection (bacteria) or infestation (parasites), might lead to **serous inflammation,** producing serous exudate, or to a **suppurative inflammation**, marked by pus formation, or even to an **ulcerative inflammation**, in which necrosis on or near the surface leads to loss of tissue and creation of a local defect (ulcer). These cases are definitely contraindicated to massage. Check with your veterinarian first.

Whatever its location, and depending on its degree of severity, an inflammation will cause from a mild pain with few overt symptoms to a very severe pain causing complete lameness. If the inflammation becomes chronic, excessive scar tissue may be formed causing more restrictions and often sustaining the inflammatory stage.

Scar Tissue Management

Following injury, inflammation, or post-surgery, the body's natural response is to develop scar tissue in that particular area to provide extra support. Scar tissue, primarily connective tissue, develops in a three dimensional way and adheres to all structures. Excess scar tissue can cause serious restrictions and pain, which in turn will lead to extra muscular compensatory tension. No scar tissue should go unevaluated, since most of the time it is associated with myofascial and muscular dysfunction.

To warm-up and loosen the area, it is best to start the treatment with regular massage therapy movements. After applying some warm hydrotherapy, use the SEW approach and then kneading movements to loosen the muscle fibers and increase circulation to the area. As a first step to break up the cross restriction caused by the scar tissue in

the fascial system, you can use gentle and deep myofascial release techniques.

To release the scar tissue, consider using the following deeper techniques. With some light kneading (thumb or finger kneading) palpate the entire scar to determine its location, and its most tender point. Evaluate thoroughly over a 360 degrees radius. Based on watching your dog's feedback signs evaluate the tenderest direction within that point. Proceed gently and carefully, in synch with the dog's feedback. The gentler you are the more responsive the dog will be. When done, loosen up the area and stir up circulation by applying gentle frictions, thumb or fingers frictions, in a circular fashion or across the fiber direction of the part being worked on.

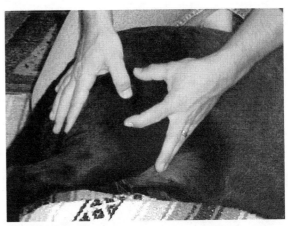

11.1 Thumb point over scar center

Next, using your thumb or finger tips, progressively apply deep pressure into the scar barrier at its most tender point, and into the direction that is most tender.

Pay attention to your dog's feedback signs, and comfort him depending on what is happen-

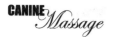

ing. Your pressure is determined by the stage of recovery and the desired effects. Start with two pounds pressure, up to five or eight pounds depending on the size of the dog and his feedback signs. Hold your pressure steadily for two to three minutes, or until you feel the release. The release is accompanied by heat and a feel of give. Once you have felt the release, progressively — not abruptly — release your pressure.

With both hands side by side, slowly apply gentle double hand friction, in a perpendicular motion to the muscle fibers, with the fingertips, and over the entire muscle, to emphasize the loosening of the fibers, and to increase the circulation to the area. You should position yourself properly, with shoulders relaxed, elbows slightly flexed, and wrist in the continuity of the forearms. Your fingers should be at ninety degrees with your hands. It is the extension-flexion movement of the fingers that produces the strumming motion.

With large dogs, use your body weight to deliver a firm pressure, between 10 to 20 pounds max, depending on the thickness of the muscle in order for this technique to be effective. Remem-

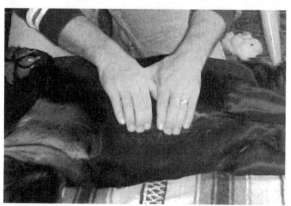

11.2 Double hand friction, back and forth

ber this deeper technique is very efficient on any scar tissue, but it is not comfortable for the dog. Be very aware and cautious, proceeding gently and progressively, comforting your dog as you proceed.

When finished, use the WES approach to thoroughly drain the area. If you suspect the dog experienced a strong release, use the "ice-cup" massage technique on the treatment area to numb the nerve endings, and control the inflammatory response. Give the area a couple of days rest before your next treatment. You can consider giving daily light massage to emphasize circulation and drainage to assist the healing. If working in coordination with a veterinarian, in a post surgery case for example, a mild anti-inflammatory can be considered after such a treatment. Check with your veterinarian,

Common Problems

Allergies — A relaxation routine will ease your dog during allergic reactions. Massaging the outside of the elbow where the biceps joins the forearm is recommended in Chinese massage.

Arthritis — Common in geriatric dogs, arthritis mostly affects the hips, lower spine, hock and knees, and to a lesser degree the shoulder and elbow. Massage won't cure arthritis, but it will help to relieve the pain and muscle tension caused by such conditions. Massage will break the "pain-tension-more-pain" cycle in the affected limb as well as the opposing limbs that bear the weight of compensation. Massage may contribute to slowing the degenerative process caused by such a condition. Try to massage early in the morning to loosen the structure involved as well as in the evening to relieve the tension buildup and the soreness. Chinese massage suggests kneading the outside of the elbow and just above and in front of the tuber calcanei on the hind leg to promote good general metabolism and fight off arthritis.

Back problems (slipped disk, sponylosis, muscle pain and spasm) — Occurring in any breed, back problems are mostly seen in the long backed dogs like Dachshunds, Beagles, Basset Hounds, Poodles, etc. The symptoms are a sudden onset of soreness/pain ranging from reluctance to get up and walk to full blown hind leg paralysis. You should first see your veterinarian to rule out nerve involvement, fractures, prolapsed disk, etc. Massage will help relieve some of the pain and muscle tension resulting from this condition on the hind legs, the forelegs, the back and neck. Focus your massage on the back region, especially the thoraco-lumbar junction area and the lumbo-sacral junction, as well as the rest of the hind legs.

Digestive problems — Do not apply a full body massage while the dog is sick. A light relaxation routine will soothe your dog. You may consider, however, a gentle kneading of the area just below the knee on the outside of the shin bone to soothe this condition as recommended in Chinese massage.

Fractures — Due to the immobilization of the limb while in the cast, there will be muscle atrophy or wasting. Massage after the cast is removed will promote muscle recovery. Massage of the other limbs and the rest of the body both before and after removal of the cast will lessen compensation tension, increase circulation, stimulate pain-releasing endorphins and comfort your dog from overall ache.

Hip dysplasia — Hip dysplasia is a fairly common problem for all breeds, but especially large, fast growing breeds of dogs. This condition is due to a poor coxofemoral joint conformation. Drugs and surgery are options for this type of problem. Massage will assist in relieving pain and compensatory muscle tension in the affected side, as well as in other areas of the body due to compensation. Focus your massage on the lower back and gluts, as well as the quadriceps and hamstring group of muscles. Try to massage early in the morning to loosen the structure involved, as well as in the evening to relieve the tension buildup and the soreness.

Luxating Patella — this condition can occur in any dog, but is most commonly seen in smaller breeds (Toy Poodles, Bichon Frise, Lhasa Apso, etc). In these breeds, the patella normally luxates medially (inside). Massage will help relieve some of the pain and compensatory muscle tension resulting from this condition. Focus your massage on the affected leg, as well as the back region due to the compensation. Any dog with luxating patellas should be evaluated by your veterinarian.

Osteochondrosis Dissecans (OCD) — This condition is common in young, fast growing, large breed dogs. It is a defect of the articular cartilage, seen mostly in the shoulder, hock, stifle and elbow. The dog will show moderate pain and lameness in the affected leg. The pain may be mild but tends to be continuous. Massage will ease the tension and pain throughout the body including both the affected and opposite limbs. Any dog with OCD must be evaluated by your veterinarian. This problem generally requires surgery.

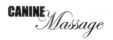

Panosteitis (growing pains) — Panosteitis is mostly seen in young, fast growing, large breed dogs. This condition involves the inflammation of the long bones in the leg and mostly occurs between the ages of six and 18 months. It shows up as a shifting lameness that affects one or more legs for a variable duration from a few days to a couple of weeks. The dog needs lots of rest and perhaps anti-inflammatory medication and diet change prescribed by your veterinarian. Massage cannot help this condition directly, but indirectly it can soothe compensation muscle tension and relax the dog of its soreness. Be cautious on the affected limb because any pressure at all on the affected bone is very painful. The rest of the body can be massaged normally.

Post surgery — Light massage will assist and promote muscle recovery as well as relax and comfort your dog. Do not work on the injury site until it is well into the chronic stage; check with your veterinarian. During convalescence, regular massage will prevent compensatory tension from developing in other muscles of the body.

Scar — Scars result from the healing of the tissues after injury. The way a scar will develop depends as much on how the body heals as it does on the original injury, or, if surgery, on the surgeon skills. Many factors can affect the severity of scarring, including the size and depth of the wound, the blood supply to the area, the thickness and color of the skin, the direction of the scar. During the chronic stage, deep friction massage technique, myofascial technique and stretching exercises can help reduce the scar formation, render it more flexible; however massage will never completely remove the scar. Only plastic surgery can reduce the size and improve the appearance of that scar if needed. See scar management earlier in this chapter.

Ununited anconeal process and fragmented coronoid process of the elbow— Both conditions, not uncommon in young dogs, require surgical correction. Massage can help during convalescence after surgery.

Massage Treatments

CHAPTER 12

The words *massage treatment* refers to a massage application over a localized body part without necessarily delivering a full body massage routine. Massage treatments are designed to deal with specific problems such as sore back, neck stiffness, and leg soreness and so on. Always apply the short version of the relaxation massage routine for a few minutes to calm and prepare your dog before starting your massage treatment.

The duration of a massage treatment varies with the situation at hand and the goals you want to achieve. In most acute situations, during the first 24 hours and when no contra-indications prevail, a treatment should last 10 to 15 minutes, or longer if the tissues are not too inflamed. It is better to repeat several shorter massage sessions over a period of several days and see consistent progressive results than taking the risk of over treating a body part and setting back the healing process by irritating and flaring up the inflammatory process. In sub-acute situations, 24 to 72 hours, the massage treatment can last from 20 to 35 minutes. In chronic situations, over 72 hours, 40 to 60 minutes is not uncommon, depending on the size of the dog.

Always keep in mind the degree of inflammation in the tissues you are massaging, the number of stress points and trigger points present and the overall state of the structure you are working on. Proceed cautiously, always checking the dog's feedback signs. Remember to use hydrotherapy to enhance the effect of your massage work. Also apply stretching exercises either during or at the end of your massage treatment to maximize the flexibility of the tissue and joints you are working on. As the dog's condition improves, follow your massage session with a mild exercise period such as walking or light trotting to complete the massage treatment, but avoid a strenuous workout.

Back Massage Treatment

Most of us have seen dogs with sore backs ranging from mild to severe, sometimes accompanied by inflammation of the muscle fibers. Usually the dog will move away from your hand when caressing or grooming his back. Sore back muscles can be a secondary condition due to the stress from painful hips especially with dogs afflicted by hip dysplasia or simply with arthritis as seen with most

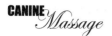

aging dogs. A sore back can also be the result of a lot of activity such as ball chasing, squirrel chasing, jumping, racing, flyball, herding, agility, pulling a harness/cart/sled, tracking and hunting. Refer to Chapter 8 for all the potential stress points in the dog's musculature.

The back muscles affected by this condition are the longissimus dorsi (SP 20 & 27), the iliocostalis (SP 21) and occasionally the serratus dorsalis thoracis (SP 5). A simple and efficient way to help your dog with this painful condition is to apply a light massage treatment before and after exercises. Place more emphasis on the massage after exercising, because warm back muscles can take a more vigorous massage that will soothe any stiffness and prevent the formation of trigger point and stress points.

After you apply the short version of the relaxation massage routine for a few minutes to calm and prepare your dog, begin your massage with a gentle application of the SEW approach with 2 to 3 pounds of pressure along the entire back, from the withers to the rump, on both sides of the spine.

Continue with several effleurages progressively increasing your pressure to 5 pounds of pressure. You might then consider using some light hacking moves (4 to 6 pounds of pressure) in order to reach deep in the muscle structure. Finish with some effleurages. Using gentle kneadings, proceed to check each of the associated stress point location (SP 5, 20, 21, 27) and treat them when necessary, using the appropriate stress point technique. If the dog appears very tender, also check SP 6, 7, 8 and 22, 23, 24, 25, 26 which are sometimes affected when severe symptoms of tension

are present in the back muscles. Apply the trigger point technique to release any trigger point that appear inflamed. Use a lot of effleurages to thoroughly drain the entire back.

Once you have checked and released all the associated stress and trigger points, gently apply finger friction along the course of the longissimus dorsi and the iliocostalis dorsi to further loosen and relax the muscle fibers. Intersperse with effleurages. Then apply the WES approach to again thoroughly drain the back area. Finish your treatment with lots of strokings over the entire back and rib cage as well as the rest of the entire body.

To enhance the effect of the massage therapy, consider hydrotherapy applications before and after your treatment. If the dog is very sore, use the ice cup massage technique or cold pack therapy to numb the nerve endings before the massage. In a more chronic phase, use warm application to loosen the fibers and stimulate circulation before the session. Also apply some stretching exercises when your massage work is done.

Neck Massage Treatment

Because the dog's neck acts as a counter weight to keep him in balance, it plays a key role in locomotion. During a sprint you will notice that the dog's head is going down when the rear legs are brought forward. The neck must be strong and flexible. This counter weight action is fundamental to the dog for him to perform smooth transitions and maintain a regular gait. Neck stiffness can restrict lateral flexion of the neck, which in turn restrict the gait. A sore neck can also be the result of a lot of activity such as ball chasing, squirrel chasing, guard dog training, obedience, pulling a harness/cart/sled, agility dog training, tracking, guide work for the visually impaired, frisbee and flyball competition.

A simple and effective way to help your dog with this condition is to use gentle massage moves over the entire neck before and after exercising. Emphasize the post exercising massage to prevent muscle stiffness. It is more beneficial to massage when the animal is warm, since the muscle can take more vigorous massage to clear away lactic acid buildup that may have developed during the workout. Familiarize yourself with the structure of the neck in order to improve your massage treatments.

The neck muscles affected by this condition are the sternocephalicus (SP 1), the splenius (SP 2), the cleidocephalicus (SP 3), the sternocephalicus (SP 4) and occasionally the rhomboideus and trapezius (SP 6, 7, 8). A simple and efficient way to help your dog with this painful condition is to apply a light massage treatment before and after exercises. Place more emphasis on the massage after exercising, because warm back muscles can take a more vigorous massage that will soothe any stiffness and prevent the formation of trigger point and stress points.

After you apply the short version of the relaxation massage routine for a few minutes to calm and prepare your dog, begin your massage with a gentle application of the SEW approach with 2 to 3 pounds of pressure along the entire neck, from the withers to the base of the base of the skull, on both sides of the spine.

Continue with several effleurages progressively increasing your pressure to 5 pounds of pressure. Using gentle kneadings, proceed to check each

of the associated stress point location (SP 1,2,3,4) and treat them when necessary, using the appropriate stress point technique. If the dog appears very tender, also check SP 6, 7, 8 and SP 5 and 9 which are sometimes affected when severe symptoms of tension are present in the neck muscles. Apply the trigger point technique to release any trigger point that appears inflamed. Use a lot of effleurages to thoroughly drain the entire neck.

Once you have checked and released all the associated stress and trigger points, gently apply finger friction along the course of the splenius, brachiocephalicus and trapezius muscles to further loosen and relax the muscle fibers. Intersperse with effleurages. Then apply the WES approach to again thoroughly drain the entire neck area. Finish your treatment with lots of strokings over the entire neck on both sides as well as the rest of the entire body.

To enhance the effect of the massage therapy, consider hydrotherapy applications before and after your treatment. If the dog is very sore, use the ice cup massage technique or cold pack therapy to numb the nerve endings before the massage. In a more chronic phase, use warm application to loosen the fibers and stimulate circulation before the session. Also apply some stretching exercises when your massage work is done.

The Forequarters Massage Treatment

The forequarters are considered to be the dog's "power steering" and play a key role in locomotion. High levels of training put a lot of physical demands on the muscles, ligaments and joints of the shoulders, chest and forelegs. Also, especially in the case of an older dog experiencing discomfort in his hindquarters, he will shift more of

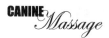

his weight to the forequarters in order to relieve the discomfort or pain in his hindquarters. If not attended to quickly, the tension in the forelegs can develop into a more serious problem, such as inflammation of the muscles fibers, or worse, the tendons or ligaments. If your dog shows signs of stiffness or discomfort in the front when turning one way or the other, this is a possible indication of tension buildup.

The forequarter muscles must be strong and flexible. If these muscles are stiff, they can restrict the entire locomotion of the foreleg, which in turn restricts the gait. Sore forequarters can be the result of a lot of activity such as ball chasing, squirrel chasing, jumping, pulling a harness/cart/sled, agility dog training, tracking, guide work for the visually impaired, frisbee and flyball competition.

A simple and effective way to help your dog with this condition is to use gentle massage moves over the entire neck before and after exercising. Emphasize the post exercising massage to prevent muscle stiffness. It is more beneficial to massage when the animal is warm, since the muscle can take more vigorous massage to clear away lactic acid buildup that may have developed during the workout. Familiarize yourself with the structure of the neck in order to improve your massage treatments.

The forequarter muscles affected by this condition are the rhomboideus and trapezius (SP 6, 7, 8), the supraspinatus and deltoideus (SP 9 & 10), the serratus ventralis thoracis (SP 11), the latissimus dorsi (SP 12) the triceps (SP 13 & 14), the pectorals (SP 15, 16 17), the extensor and flexor muscles (SP 18 & 19) and occasionally the serratus dorsalis thoracis (SP 5) and longissimus dorsi

(SP 20). A simple and efficient way to help your dog with this painful condition is to apply a light massage treatment before and after exercises. Place more emphasis on the massage after exercising, because warm back muscles can take a more vigorous massage that will soothe any stiffness and prevent the formation of trigger point and stress points.

After you apply the short version of the relaxation massage routine for a few minutes to calm and prepare your dog, begin your massage with a gentle application of the SEW approach with 2 to 3 pounds of pressure along the entire forequarter, from the top of the shoulder to the paw. Continue with several effleurages progressively increasing to 5 pounds of pressure. Using gentle kneadings, proceed to check each of the associated stress point location (SP 6 to 19) and treat them when necessary, using the stress point technique. If the dog appears very tender, also check SP 5 and SP 20 which are sometimes affected when severe symptoms of tension are present in the neck muscles. Apply the trigger point technique to release any trigger point that appears inflamed. Use a lot of effleurages to thoroughly drain the entire neck.

Once you have checked and released all the associated stress and trigger points, gently apply finger friction along the course of the trapezius, rhomboideus, supraspinatus, deltoideus and the extensor and flexor muscles to further loosen and relax the muscle fibers. Intersperse with effleurages. Then apply the WES approach to again thoroughly drain the entire neck area.

Finish your treatment with lots of stroking over the entire forequarter. Duplicate the same treatment on the other leg. When done, use stroking over the rest of the entire body. To enhance the effect of the massage therapy, consider hydrotherapy applications before and after your treatment. If the dog is very sore, use the ice cup massage technique or cold pack therapy to numb the nerve endings before the massage. In a more chronic phase, use warm application to loosen the fibers and stimulate circulation before the session. Also apply some stretching exercises when your massage work is done.

The Hindquarters Massage Treatment

The hindquarters are considered to be the dog's "engine" and play a key role in locomotion. High levels of playing or training put a lot of physical demands on the muscles, ligaments and joints of the hips and hind legs. He may show extra muscle tension due to the soreness created by arthritis in his joints. If not attended to quickly, the tension in the hind legs can develop into a more serious problem, such as inflammation of the muscle fibers, or worse, the tendons or ligaments. If your dog shows signs of stiffness or discomfort in the hindquarters when turning one way or the other, this is a possible indication of tension buildup.

The hindquarter muscles must be strong and flexible. If these muscles are stiff it can restrict the entire locomotion of the hind leg, which in turn restricts the gait. Sore hindquarters can be the result of a lot of activity such as ball chasing, squirrel chasing, agility dog training, pulling a harness/cart/sled, hunting, tracking, guard dog training, herding, racing frisbee and flyball competition.

A simple and effective way to help your dog with this condition is to use gentle massage moves over the entire hindquarter before and after exercising. Emphasize the post exercising massage to prevent muscle stiffness. It is more beneficial to massage when your dog is warm, since the muscle can take more vigorous massage to clear any potential stress points and also trigger points from the lactic acid buildup that develop during the workout. Familiarize yourself with the structure of the hindquarters in order to improve your massage treatments.

The hindquarter muscles affected by this condition are the gluteals (SP 27,38), the biceps femoris (SP 28 & 29), the semitendinosus and semimembranosus (SP 34 & 35), the TFL and iliopsoas (SP 36 & 37), the vastus lateralis and rectus femoris (SP 31 & 32), the gastrocnemius (SP 30), the adductors (SP 33), the extensor and flexor muscles (SP 39 & 40) and occasionally the abdominals (SP 22 to 25) and back muscles (SP 5, 20 & 27). A simple and efficient way to help your dog with this painful condition is to apply a light massage treatment before and after exercises. Place more emphasis on the massage after exercising, because warm back muscles can take a more vigorous massage that will soothe any stiffness and prevent the formation of trigger point and stress points.

After you apply the short version of the relaxation massage routine for a few minutes to calm and prepare your dog, begin your massage with a gentle application of the SEW approach with 2 to 3 pounds of pressure along the entire hindquarters, from the hip to the paw. Continue with several effleurages increasing progressively your pressure to 5 pounds of pressure. Using gentle kneadings, proceed to check each of the associated stress point location (SP 27 to 40) and treat them when necessary, using the stress point tech-

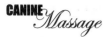

nique. If the dog appears very tender, also check SP 20 to 26 which are sometimes affected when severe symptoms of tension are present in the neck muscles. Apply the trigger point technique to release any trigger point that appears inflamed. Use a lot of effleurages to thoroughly drain the entire hindquarters.

Once you have checked and released all the associated stress and trigger points, gently apply finger friction along the course of the entire muscle groups including the gluts, hamstrings, quads and lower leg muscles to further loosen and relax the muscle fibers. Intersperse with effleurages. Then apply the WES approach to again thoroughly drain the entire hindquarters area. Duplicate the same treatment on the other leg. When you are finished use lots of stroking over the entire hindquarters and the rest of the entire body.

To enhance the effect of the massage therapy, consider hydrotherapy applications before and after your treatment. If the dog is very sore, use the ice cup massage technique or cold pack therapy to numb the nerve endings before the massage. In a more chronic phase, use warm application to loosen the fibers and stimulate circulation before the session. Also apply some stretching exercises when your massage work is done.

Conclusion

These four treatment outlines were given to you for guidance in your canine massage education. With practice you will become familiar with each course of treatment and soon will discover what works best for you. Remember to insure that no contraindications apply, and to check with your veterinarian for the best course of action.

Massage Recommendations for Dog Breeds and Activities

CHAPTER

13

This chapter contains a list of the 100 most common breeds of dog in North America and the areas to emphasize during a massage. Because a large number of dogs are of mixed breed, go through the list and choose the breed(s) that best matches your dog's body type. For example, if you have a short-legged hound with a long back, then referring to the Basset Hound breed listing would be appropriate.

Always remember, before you begin massaging your dog, ensure there are no contraindications. Should undiagnosed symptoms arise, please contact your veterinarian.

Always start your massage with a relaxation massage routine. Continue with a maintenance massage routine and emphasize the areas listed below, according to your dog's breed.

Breed	Weight (approx) in lbs.	Areas to Emphasis With Massage
Afghan Hound	50-60	neck, shoulders, back
Airedale	45-50	hind quarters, hip area
Akita	75-85	back, hind quarters
Alaskan Malamute	75-85	hind quarters, hip area
American Bulldog	60-120	shoulders, chest, hind quarters
Australian Cattle dog	30-50	neck, chest, hind quarters
Australian Shepherd	40-50	lower back, hip area
Basenji	20-23	hips & flanks
Basset Hound	40-55	neck, entire back, limbs

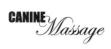

Breed	Weight (approx) in lbs.	Areas to Emphasis With Massage
Beagle	20-35	neck, shoulders, back
Bearded Collie	40-60	neck, back
Bedlington Terrier	25-40	neck, back, abdomen
Belgian Sheepdog	40-55	neck, back, hind quarters, hips
Bernese Mountain Dog	60-80	back, hip area
Bichon Frise	12-20	neck, back
Bloodhound	60-80	neck, back
Border Collie	40-50	neck, shoulders, lower back
Border Terrier	12-14	hips, hind quarters, stifles
Borzoi	75-105	neck, back, hip area
Boston Terrier	15-25	shoulders, chest, back
Bouvier	80-110	shoulders, neck, hind quarters
Boxer	50-70	neck, back, hind quarters
Brittany Spaniel	25-40	back
Bull Terrier	40-60	neck, lower back and hips
Cairn Terrier	20-30	jaw, neck, back, hips, flanks
Cavalier King Charles Spaniel	10-20	back, hips
Chesapeake Bay Retriever	55-75	back, hind quarters
Chihuahua	2-6	neck, shoulders, hind quarters, stifles
Chow Chow	50-60	back, hind quarters, stifles
Cocker Spaniel	20-30	neck, back, hip area
Collie	40-65	back, hips, flanks, abdomen
Dachshund	10-25	neck, back, hips, hind quarters
Dalmatian	40-45	back, hind quarters
Doberman Pinscher	50-70	back, foreleg, shoulders, hind quarters
English Bulldog	40-50	neck, chest, back
English Setter	50-70	shoulders, back, hind quarters
English Springer Spaniel	25-50	back, hind quarters

Breed	Weight (approx) in lbs.	Areas to Emphasis With Massage
English Toy Spaniels	9-12	back, hind quarters
Finnish Spitz	50-80	neck, chest, back
Flat-Coated Retriever	60-70	back, hind quarters
Fox Hound	30-50	neck, back
Fox Terrier	17-20	neck, shoulders, lower back
French Bulldog	22-28	back, chest, hips
German Shepherd	60-85	back, hip area
German Shorthaired Pointer	45-70	back, hind quarters
Golden Retriever	55-75	neck, back, hip area
Gordon Setter	60-80	shoulders, back, hind quarters
Great Dane	100-150	back, hip area, hind quarters
Great Pyrenees	80-110	back, hind quarters
Greyhound	60-70	neck, withers, back, hip area
Griffon	15-35	neck, shoulders, back
Hovawart	66-88	back, hind quarters
Irish Setter	45-70	forelegs, shoulders, back
Irish Wolfhound	80-110	back, hip area, hind quarters
Jack Russel Terrier	10-20	back, hind quarters
Keeshond	30-40	back, hind quarters
Kerry Blue Terrier	30-40	back, hind quarters
Labrador Retriever	55-75	forelegs, back, hip area
Lakeland Terrier	15-20	chest, back, hind quarters
Leonberger	90-120	back, hind quarters
Lhasa Apso	10-15	back, abdomen
Maltese	5-7	back
Mastiff	90-150	neck, back, hind quarters
Newfoundland	120-150	back, hip area, hind quarters
Norwegian Elkhound	40-60	neck, back, hind quarters

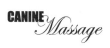
Breed	Weight (approx) in lbs.	Areas to Emphasis With Massage
Nova Scotia Duck Tolling Retriever	35-50	back, hind quarters
Old English Sheepdog	80-100	neck, back, hind quarters
Papillon	8-15	neck, back
Pekingese	10-14	neck, back
Pomeranian	3-7	neck, shoulders, hind legs
Poodle (miniature)	12-25	neck, shoulders, back, hind legs
Poodle (standard)	35-50	foreleg, back & hip area
Poodle (toy)	12-15	neck, back, hind quarters
Portuguese Water Dog	35-60	forelegs, back, hind quarters
Pug	14-18	neck, back, hind leg
Rhodesian Ridgeback	55-65	back, hind quarters
Rottweiler	95-120	back, hip area
Saint Bernard	100-200	lower back, hips, hind legs
Saluki	45-60	hip area, hind quarters
Samoyed	35-60	back, hind quarters
Schnauzer (giant)	70-90	shoulders, back, hind quarters
Schnauzer (miniature)	12-15	neck, flank, hind quarters
Schnauzer (standard)	35-55	back, hind quarters
Scottish Terrier	18-22	neck, back, hind quarters
Shetland Sheepdog	20-35	back, hind quarters
Shih Tzu	12-20	neck, back, hind quarters
Siberian Husky	35-60	neck, back, hind quarters
Vizsla	50-65	neck, back, hind quarters
Weimaraner	60-80	back, flanks, hind quarters
Welsh Corgi	15-25	neck, shoulders, back, hind quarters
Welsh Terrier	15-25	neck, hind quarters
West Highland White Terrier	12-20	neck, jaw, back, flanks, hind quarters
Wheaten Terrier	30-40	back, hind quarters
Whippet	15-25	shoulder, back, hind quarters
Yorkshire Terrier	4-7	back, hind quarters

Activities

An active dog is a complete enjoyment of both dog and owner. Like human athlete, an active dog will develop extra muscular tension as a result of the increased activity.

Here are a variety of activities and the corresponding areas of tension that should be emphasized during a massage.

Remember, all muscle groups work at once and you will find more than one area of muscular tension. In Chapter 8, you are given an outline of the most common stress areas found in active dogs, and a "trouble-spots" massage routine to keep the muscular stress to a minimum. Regular massage will ensure the good fitness and top performance of your dog.

Activities	Areas Of Muscular Tension
Agility	chest, forelegs, back, hind quarters
Den Trials	neck, back, hind quarters
Draft Dog	neck, shoulders, chest, back, hind quarters
Field Trials Pointers	neck, shoulders, back
Field Trials Retrivers	neck, shoulders, back, limbs
Fly Ball	neck, back, hind quarters
Frisbee Catching	neck, forelegs, back, hind quarters
Scent Hurdle Dog	neck, back, hind quarters
Schutzhund	neck, shoulders, chest, back, hip area,limbs
Sledding	neck, shoulders, chest, back, limbs
Stockdogs	neck, back, limbs
Tracking	neck, shoulders, chest
Water Rescue	neck, shoulders, chest, limbs

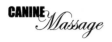

Keeping Records

CHAPTER 14

Especially for those who are doing canine massage professionally, keeping records of your massage work and the findings after each massage treatment should be considered as important as keeping records of veterinarian visits.

Your records should contain the following:

- History and background information (to the best of your knowledge) on the dog. For example, previous ownership, past accidents or injuries, type of training, if applicable.
- Personality traits like playfulness, shyness, hyperactivity, calmness, nastiness when in cage, biting, etc.
- Medication(s), if any.
- Type of training the dog is involved in at the present time, plus his tendencies during training, like problems with bending, jumping, or galloping, etc.
- Notes on the overall condition of your dog at the time of each massage. List the various stress points, trigger points, inflammations, swellings, if any, and the finding of your 4 T's.
- Whenever the dog gets hurt, record what happened, how and when, as well as the location of the injury on the dog. Also note what treatment was given at the time.

- When using equipment on your dog (for example, a harness), record when and how the dog responded to the change over the following seven to 10 days.

This information will help you appreciate the progress of your dog following your massage treatments. By keeping thorough notes, you will have a clear idea of any changes in the symptoms shown by your dog. It will also help you provide better feedback to your veterinarian.

Good records also give you feedback on the impact of your training program and changes in the dog's life (for example, traveling, competitions, new home, etc.).

In illustration 14.1, there is an example of the case study we take with each dog we work on.

Knowing your dog well will assist you in determining the best maintenance massage program. With the practice of regular massage, you will be more aware of signs and symptoms which tell you when your dog needs veterinary attention, much sooner than with the usual practice of grooming. You will never look at or touch your dog the same way again.

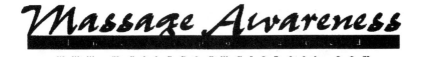

www.massageawareness.com

CASE - STUDY

Name:	**Cleopatra**	Owner:	**Brigitte Hawkins**
Breed:	**Black Lab**	Address:	**3856 Peachtree Lane**
Color:	**Black**	Tel:	**561 888 8245**
Size:	**22inches**	Vet:	**Banfield Vets**
Weight:	**58 lbs**	Tel:	**561 974 2356**
Markings:	**None**	Trainer:	**B. Hawkins**
Age:	**3 years**	Tel:	**561 888 8245**
Groom:	**PetsMart**	Tel:	
Discipline:	**Obedience, Agility, Tracking**		

Conditioning: ☐≤ Low   ☐≤ Moderate   ☐P High   ☐≤ Overweight   ☐≤ Underweight

Major complaint: What, Where, When, How...   **Shortness   of   stride   in   the   protraction**

movement of the left hind leg when

warming up. After training definite lameness appears on the same leg.

History of present illness: **Same problem six months ago, comes and goes.**

History of past illness: **N/A**

Massage Awareness Inc. offers canine massage services to assist people who wish to promote the wellness of their dog. The information provided during the massage is for educational purposes. The services of M.A. Inc. are not intended as a substitute for the medical advice of a licensed veterinarian. This is not a medical treatment directed at a specific physical dysfunction. The dog owner should always consult a veterinarian in matters relating to the health of the animal. M.A. Inc. asks you to indicated below, by signing this paper, that you have read an understood this statement and that you will take full responsibility for this choice. M.A. Inc. shall not be held responsible for any damage or injury resulting from massages services. The undersigned hereby releases and agree to indemnify and save harmless the corporation of Massage Awareness Inc., their representative officers, employees, volunteers or agents, from any claims, costs, expenses of whatsoever kind or nature for loss, injury or damage to person, animal or property howsoever caused arising from massage services.

I, the undersigned, have read the above and voluntarily agree to provide this waiver and indemnity.

Brigitte Hawkins	**Brigitte Hawkins**	**May 14, 2003**
(Signature)	(Print name)	(Date)

14.1a Example of page one of Case Study (filled out).

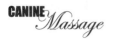
Preliminary   **Good overall, no inflammation present. Strong muscle tone in the**

Evaluation: **neck (brachiocefalicus, splenius) on the right side of the neck**

Shoulder muscles are tight (rhomboid, trapezius, spinalis dorsi) especially on the right

side. Back muscles are tight along the lumbar area. The gluteal and hamstring muscle

groups show high tone, especially on the right. Soreness upon palpation of the

sacroiliac joint, especially on the left side. Legs are good and flexible upon massage

and stretching.

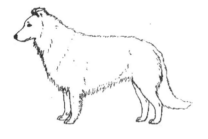
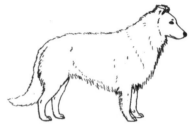

❏ P Relaxation Massage Routine   ❏ ≤ Myofascial Massage Routine
❏ P 40StressPoint Check-up   ❏ ≤ Lymph Drainage Massage Routine
❏ P Full Body Maint. Massage Routine   ❏ P Stretching Legs & Neck
❏ ≤ Sport Massage Routine   ❏ P Referred to Vet P Chiro - Acupunture

Comments: **The muscular tension found on the right side is mostly compen-**
satory muscle tension, secondary to the jammed left sacroiliac joint. We recommend
supervision by veterinarian before going back to training and further therapy.

Maintenance Program: **No running exercise until authorized by a veterinarian.**
Daily application of hydrotherapy (vascular flush) over the sacrum area, followed by
gentle full body massage and stretching exercise.

Massage Awareness, Inc.
Town Square at Wellington, 11924 Forest Hill Blvd, Suite 22-102, Wellington, FL 33414 USA
Tel: 561 – 383 8205 / Fax: 561 – 383 8206 / Cell: 561 523 3608

14.1b   Example of page two of Case Study (filled out).

Massage Awareness

w w w . m a s s a g e a w a r e n e s s . c o m

CASE - STUDY

Name: _____	Owner: _____
Breed: _____	Address: _____
Color: _____	Tel: _____
Size: _____	Vet: _____
Weight: _____	Tel: _____
Markings: _____	Trainer: _____
Age: _____	Tel: _____
Groom: _____	Tel: _____
Discipline: _____	

Conditioning: ☐≤ Low   ☐≤ Moderate   ☐P High   ☐≤ Overweight   ☐≤ Underweight

Major complaint: What, Where, When, How... _____

_____

_____

History of present illness: _____

_____

_____

History of past illness: _____

Massage Awareness Inc. offers canine massage services to assist people who wish to promote the wellness of their dog. The information provided during the massage is for educational purposes. The services of M.A. Inc. are not intended as a substitute for the medical advice of a licensed veterinarian. This is not a medical treatment directed at a specific physical dysfunction. The dog owner should always consult a veterinarian in matters relating to the health of the animal. M.A. Inc. asks you to indicated below, by signing this paper, that you have read an understood this statement and that you will take full responsibility for this choice. M.A. Inc. shall not be held responsible for any damage or injury resulting from massages services. The undersigned hereby releases and agree to indemnify and save harmless the corporation of Massage Awareness Inc., their representative officers, employees, volunteers or agents, from any claims, costs, expenses of whatsoever kind or nature for loss, injury or damage to person, animal or property howsoever caused arising from massage services.
I, the undersigned, have read the above and voluntarily agree to provide this waiver and indemnity.

_____   _____   _____
(Signature)   (Print name)   (Date)

14.2a Example of page one of Case Study (blank).

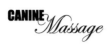

Preliminary Evaluation: _____

_____

_____

_____

_____

_____

- ☐ ≤ Relaxation Massage Routine
- ☐ ≤ 40StressPoint Check-up
- ☐ ≤ Full Body Maint. Massage Routine
- ☐ ≤ Sport Massage Routine

- ☐ ≤ Myofascial Massage Routine
- ☐ ≤ Lymph Drainage Massage Routine
- ☐ ≤ Stretching Legs & Neck
- ☐ ≤ Referred to Vet – Chiro - Acupunture

Comments: _____

_____

_____

_____

Maintenance Program: _____

_____

_____

Massage Awareness, Inc.
Town Square at Wellington, 11924 Forest Hill Blvd, Suite 22-102, Wellington, FL 33414 USA
Tel: 561 – 383 8205 / Fax: 561 – 383 8206 / Cell: 561 523 3608

14.2b Example of page two of Case Study (blank).

RECOMMENDED READING

There are lots of great books on the subject of canine health and fitness. Here are few of my favorites. Most of the following titles are available from Dogwise at 1-800-776-2665 or www.dogwise.com

Agility Training–The Fun Sport for All Dogs, Jane Simmons-Moake, 1991
For both the casual and highly competitive agility enthusiast. Includes obstacle construction plans.

An Atlas of Animal Anatomy for Artists, 2nd Edition, Revised & Expanded, W. Ellenberger, H. Baum and H. Dittrich, 1990
288 life-like drawings of animals show in detailed full view and beneath-the-skin drawings of musculature. Contains plenty of accurate canine muscle charts.

Canine Massage Video, A Visual Guide, Jean-Pierre Hourdebaigt.
The perfect companion to *Canine Massage, A Complete Reference Manual.* 90 minutes demonstrating all the principles and techniques discussed in the book.

Canine Physical Therapy: Orthopedic Physical Therapy, Deborah M. Gross-Saunders, M.S.P.T., O.C.S., 2002
A basic overview of physical therapy procedures including anatomy, biomechanics, mechanisms of injury, and treatment principles. Well illustrated.

Dogsteps, A New Look, Rachel Page Elliott, 2001
This is a must! Educates anyone interested in canine conformation and gait. Aids the reader in identifying and understanding good and faulty gait.

Dogsteps, What to Look for in a Dog (Video), Rachel Page Elliott, 1986
See rare moving x-ray photographs of the dog in motion. Dogs with correct and incorrect gait are shown with narrative from experts. 68 minutes.

Four Paws, Five Directions: A Guide to Chinese Medicine for Cats and Dogs, Cheryl Schwartz, D.V.M., 1996
Chinese medicine and how it relates to dogs. Acupuncture, food and herbs and how they relate to dogs.

Introduction to Dog Agility, Margaret H. Bonham, 2000
Written for the beginner, this manual covers all aspects of the sport including valuating fitness, beginning training, learning the obstacles and more. Full-color illustrations.

Jumping from A to Z, M. Christine Zink D.V.M., Ph.D., and Julie Daniels, 1996
Mechanics of canine jump training, a complete jump training program, conditioning for jumping. Specific training for obedience, agility and flyball.

Miller's Guide To The Dissection Of The Dog, 5th Edition, Howard Evans, Ph.D. and Alexander deLahunta, D.V.M., Ph.D., 2000
In-depth information on the canine muscle groups and other structures. A veterinary textbook.

Peak Performance, Coaching the Canine Athlete, M. Christine Zink D.V.M., Ph.D., 1997
Selecting, conditioning, and coaching the canine athlete. Prevention, rehabilitation, problem solving.

Physical Therapy for the Canine Athlete, Suzanne Clothier & Sue Ann Lesser, D.V.M., 1996
Handy booklet that explains physical therapy techniques to help the dog recover from injuries.

Index